Health
for
Godly
Generations

A Reformational Perspective

Health
for
Godly
Generations

Renée DeGroot

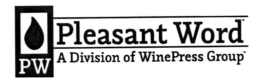
Pleasant Word
A Division of WinePress Group
PW

Pleasant Word (a division of WinePress Publishing, PO Box 428, Enumclaw, WA 98022) functions only as book publisher. As such, the ultimate design, content, editorial accuracy, and views expressed or implied in this work are those of the author.

Nothing written in this book may be construed as professional health advice and neither the author nor publisher is liable for the understanding or practice of anything written herein.

Unless otherwise noted, all Scriptures are taken from the *King James Version* of the Bible.

ISBN 13: 978-1-4141-1603-7
ISBN 10: 1-4141-1603-9
Library of Congress Catalog Card Number: 2009909163

Dedicated to my mother Laura, my brother Bryce, and my sister-in-law Sarah. As our family grows, may it increase in godliness, healthfulness, and victorious living for Christ's Kingdom.

Written in memory of my late father, Mark DeGroot, who, in a journal he wrote to me, recommended that I should direct my efforts toward becoming a writer—the dream pursuit of my youth, which he encouraged.

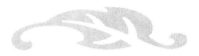

Contents

Rising in the morning,
a family breakfasts on the most popular,
most convenient foods,
filling themselves up with little contemplation.
Thirty years after, the parents and children
are riddled with disease,
have lessened ability to perform their work,
and wonder how this ever happened.
Sixty years previous, their grandparents
ate the whole foods of nature and thrived—
but never put this practice into words
or passed it down...

Rising in the morning,
the sun shines on God's abundant earth,
alive with plants and animals
and the crown of creation—men and women.
Fifty years after, the production of chemicals
has left an indelible scar
in the soil, in the sea, and in the sky.
Ninety years previous, the landscape
was so pure and clean, that people
did not consider if polluting it
would ever matter...

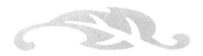

Acknowledgments

GRATITUDE IS OWED to numerous people who provided assistance, whether tangible service, audible encouragement, or useful instruction. God orchestrated relationships and brought information to my attention at such needful times and in such a perfect order that I am continually amazed by His providence.

My mother, Laura DeGroot, gave frequent advice regarding the fundamental content of my manuscript and graciously supported the time I have spent writing and the necessary decisions to be made. She lovingly cooked many meals for the two of us while I stayed at my desk working right up until lunchtime...and dinnertime...and again after dinner. My brother, Bryce DeGroot, gave counsel from his wide knowledge of economics and entrepreneurship, and has been an invaluable listener for any type of question I have had. He's been my best friend for as long as I can remember. My sister-in-law, Sarah DeGroot, spent countless hours as a new wife editing each chapter—applying her expertise in English grammar and making me clarify ambiguous concepts. It is a privilege to be related to her and her Texas family.

I want to thank Molly Gregory, a certified massage therapist who is training to be a natural health consultant, and Lydia Hayden, a registered nurse, for their dear friendship and their willingness to critique my manuscript. Many conversations with my chiropractor, Dr. Kimberly Anderson, influenced my thinking about medical care and the historical evidence for healthful diets—not to mention that her chiropractic care has helped me significantly. Correspondence with fellow home school author Natalie Wickham has given helpful direction to my intentions for sharing my message. Among many treasured lessons she has taught me, Kathryn Lundberg first introduced me to alternative diets and inspired me by her efforts to cook nutritiously when her healing depended on it. These ladies, as well as many others, have helped to shape and sharpen my beliefs about health and my desire to share them with the Christian community. Not only discussions, but dining in the homes of friends over the years has been some of the greatest education and motivation of all.

I also wish to acknowledge several of the numerous men whose ministries and publications have helped to develop my worldview: Douglas Phillips and Dr. Joe Morecraft III and what they so passionately teach about transforming culture according to the Word of God; Dr. Paul Jehle and Kevin Swanson and what they so victoriously teach about distinctive Christian education; Dr. Jordan Rubin and Joel Salatin and their courageous leadership in the advancement of traditional, nourishing food; and Pastors Bryan Clark and Jeff Hamling of Gallatin Valley Presbyterian Church and what they so clearly teach about the glory of God and the gospel of Jesus Christ.

Working with Adam Cothes and the Pleasant Word division of WinePress Publishing has been an excellent experience and one I would easily recommend. They provided all the services a new author could want, and their communication was always accommodating, personable, and professional. I am thankful for their work in designing the beautiful book you now hold from the plain document once dormant on my computer.

The nature photographs interspersed throughout the book are used with permission of Emily Elizabeth Case (after chapters 2, 14, 17, 24, and 26) as well as another Southern young lady who wishes to remain anonymous.

To the friends, acquaintances, and future readers not mentioned by name—it is you whose quiet faithfulness in purchasing wholesome food, feeding your family nutritiously, and maintaining a healthy home will change the world whether or not it ever brings acclaim.

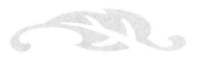

Introduction

"Beloved, I wish above all things that thou mayest prosper
and be in health, even as thy soul prospereth."
—3 John 1:2

*H*EALTH: THE STATE of wholesome well-being; the flourishing condition of the body; freedom from physical disease. With regard to etymology, the Old English word *hāl* and the Indo-European *kailo-* are the roots from which *hale, healthy, whole,* and *holy,* are all derived.[1] Health is not only the best condition for our bodies to be in, but it leads to a beautiful, hale, and hearty complexion and constitution. Health is synonymous with wholeness, or, the completeness that God created in us; it relates to holiness, because the state of our body and spirit do and should influence one another.

People who want to enjoy a state of wellness and goodness will pursue it in exceedingly different ways. The holistic approach seeks the health of the unified whole, consisting of mind, spirit, and body. Various humanistic practices pursue the naturalness of the body and the elements of nature above anything else. Some people believe that whatever is offered for sale at the grocer will sufficiently nourish them. Other people think that they are quite healthy—until they become ill. To many people, modern medicine is the most advanced yet and offers the best answers available.

For the thoughtful Christian, none of these reactions are prudent. We must seek, as in all areas of life, the wisdom from God's Word, the knowledge from history, and an understanding of the times. Christians must analyze the philosophies in the world around them and be involved in harnessing the elements of God's creation to use in His service.

My purpose in *Health for Godly Generations* is not to give an ultimate diet prescription. I have been studying the facts and history of health and nutrition for only several years. After learning from the writing of many astute men and women—leaders in their field—I have little innovative to say except in application to the Christian life. I seek to synthesize the available information enough to make it palatable to those people not previously interested in nutrition. Scientific discoveries and studies are always being made, and more Christians should be involved; however, sufficient persuasive data exists, if only we would express concern and interest. My purpose is to apply godly principles to this important area of our lives and to promote awareness regarding the repercussions of our dietary choices. I trust that referring to numerous recognized authorities in the field of nutrition will give credence to the principles I offer and will encourage the reader to refer to their work for additional research.

If certain foods are "healthful" and some are utterly not, a standard must be determined and a line must be drawn. Raising a standard is an essential of Christianity, in which faith we are called not to ride the line, vacillating between the flesh and the spirit or between worldliness and righteousness. God desires passion more than apathy, as He told the Laodicean church in the book of Revelation, when He preferred that they were either cold or hot instead of lukewarm (Rev. 3:15).

Being an American with many choices and opportunities of food to consume, and many conflicting suggestions from media about what contributes to health, has influenced the angle from which I share. I write to you as part of a younger generation—the generation which approached adulthood at the turn of the twenty-first century. My generation is simultaneously *removed* from the generation of our grandparents, when life was arguably simpler, and *bombarded* with the recent technological "progress" which leaves short-sighted evidence as to the effects of these new developments. Undeniably, health problems are around us; now is the time to think like Christians for the glory of God and the benefit of His temples, our bodies. Unlike the opinion of some medical practitioners, health *is* directly linked to food consumption and other lifestyle factors. Only in the previous century has the prevalence of degenerative diseases and newfangled foods risen noticeably and simultaneously.

I have written this book primarily for Christian families who desire to start considering their health and for those who desire that their lives are pleasing to their Creator and Savior—though they may have seldom thought about health. I plan to give principles to support the inclinations of those who are already journeying toward vital health. I have many friends in both categories. My hope is that this book will provide my readers with "food for thought"—with reasons for living healthfully and a few resources for doing so. My wish is that this book will introduce my readers to a whole world of opportunities and information and will encourage further study of this subject.

To accomplish these goals, I will speak first about a few things Christians ought to believe and then look at living out these beliefs in a healthful lifestyle. I want to take the best things Christians believe about God, creation, and the Bible, and get "down to earth" with them—applying these beliefs to the most common things people do, including eating and taking care of ourselves. What better way is there to appreciate God's world than by healthy bodies giving glory to their Maker for the wisdom of His plan?

As a side note, I chose the subtitle of "a Reformational perspective" for a reason. My family greatly respects the faith and spirit of the Protestant Reformers of five hundred years ago and the lessons that their lives have taught us. Three main themes that I use in my exposition have been informed by a study of the great Reformers. These men were passionate about submitting to and applying the whole and authoritative counsel of Scripture in every area of life. They believed in the importance of evaluating God's work in history, and they followed in the steps of other wise and godly men, the leaders who had gone before them. Also, the Reformers worked laboriously for the next generation, making sacrifices so that their progeny could have more liberty to obey God, and leaving a legacy of instruction so that future generations would be prompted toward godliness. Scripture, theology, history, teaching, learning, and successive generations all featured prominently in the era of the Protestant Reformation, and the same factors pertain to strong Christian culture in any time period including ours today. For that reason, the above themes have a deliberate place in my discussion of healthfulness.

My understanding is that written words are one of the finest ways to give weight and endurance to a message which otherwise might not be heard from a young woman. I seek to address the area of Christian health because I know it is being undermined on many fronts and is strongly attacked by the world; this issue is more than just an "interest." As I write in challenging political and economic times, I am aware that physical nutrition might not be foremost on people's minds. However, I believe that every thought must be taken captive for Christ as He gives ability, without procrastinating for a better time or waiting for more experience. In the following pages, I try to address what is the big picture surrounding our health as well as additional issues that influence health—the political and economic scenes. I hope this book is an inspiration for you to serve God with a vigorous life, more so than simply an impetus for distinguishing between butter and margarine.

In the following study, I want this verse to be earnestly employed: "Whether therefore ye eat, or drink, or whatsoever ye do, do all to the glory of God" (1 Cor. 10:31).

May our health ever be reformed as it trails behind the reformation in our hearts.

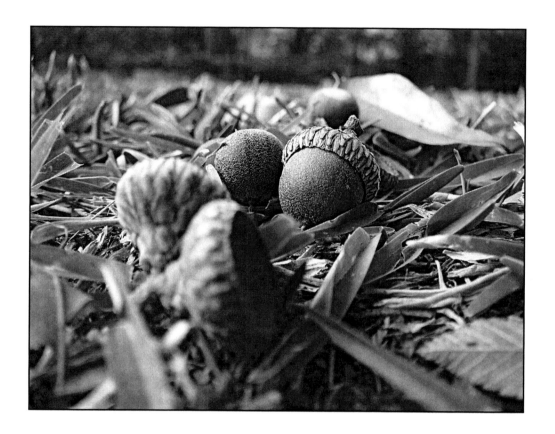

Chapter One

God Created All Things

"What joy to discern the minute in infinity!
The vast to perceive in the small, what divinity!"[1]

—Jakob Bernoulli

In the beginning God created the heaven and the earth...And God saw every thing that he had made, and, behold, it was very good. And the evening and the morning were the sixth day.

—Genesis 1:1, 31

The creature itself also shall be delivered from the bondage of corruption into the glorious liberty of the children of God. For we know that the whole creation groaneth and travaileth in pain together until now.

—Romans 8:21, 22

DISCERNING THE CORRELATION between the philosophical concept of "the One and the Many" has been an ancient enigma. Why does the fact that oranges grow in tropical climates have anything to do with the fact that oats grow in cold climates? How can one source undergird all things, including seemingly schizophrenic details? The Almighty Jehovah God provides the only answer to this problem. His Word tells us He is the Creator of all things in heaven and earth, and that He created all things out of nothing in six literal days [see Appendix A for elaboration]. Each aspect of creation was created to be very good, yet man's sin has affected the whole universe. Creation would deteriorate without God's upholding sustenance. The outlook on earth would be hopeless without the incarnation of Jesus Christ, who transforms His people and commands them to subdue the earth. The whole creation groans and travails while the Lord Almighty uses it as His stage for saving and sanctifying His Church. All creation will continue in this way until Christ's return when He will create a "new heavens and new earth."

The One True God created many facets of beauty. One word, sin, has affected it all. Elements of weather, as necessary as they are, are often destructive. Mankind, created in the image of God, can have physical disorders. What can unify the facts that one fruit tree grows to be a beautiful specimen, but another crop is attacked by devastating insects? How can this man feel perfectly healthy, but this woman struggle with an illness? I would submit that the glory of God is the unifying factor. He decrees all things to proclaim, eventually, the honor of His name. Insofar as God gives grace, mankind is commanded to perform all actions for the glory of God's name.

Climates and seasonal cycles have changed since the worldwide flood sent by God in Noah's time. Prior to that great flood, mankind was forever cursed with struggling to harvest the fruit of the earth. Through cultivating the earth and subduing it, man can never change the harsh conditions that God allows in our environment, but man can take joy in doing what God created humanity to do. However imperfectly man may labor on the earth in obedience to God, the earth still praises her Creator.

People see no contradiction between saying Jesus is their Creator and Lord and then going on to fill their bodies with artificial junk. I submit that the principle of the "one and the many" gives unity to seemingly separate facts, and ties these facts together so that they cannot be divided. Jesus is Lord of our physical bodies and our diets just as He is Lord spiritually over our souls and, broadly, over the whole universe. To divide any aspect of life into a "neutral" or "secular" realm is to say that Jesus is not Lord over some realms and that we do not care whether we obey Him there.

Have human bodies evolved and progressed to the ability to eat newfangled "foods"? Hardly. Our physical bodies are the same as God created them—but our food is usually not, having been altered. Our bodies are letting us know that they can only endure altered input for so long before giving out. Biological evolution, a theory radically opposed to the testimony of Scripture, is not to be accepted and therefore provides no basis for the "evolution" of foods beyond their original design. We were created fearfully and wonderfully by God Himself, as was the rest of creation. Plants and animals, seas and skies, men and women, were all created "very good." Adam and Eve's first sin was eating what God told them not to, and people have been falling into the same temptation for the last six thousand years. People are not satisfied with what God said or with what He created, seeking rather to enhance their diets according to fleshly wisdom. The inclination to alter and adulterate natural foods is sliding deeper into disobedience, not scaling a ladder of so-called progress.

If we have faith in God and repent of sin, He will give the grace to obey and to follow our Creator and Savior. What does He redeem us from if not from depravity and sin? Christians are saved to live a victorious life of obedience. Except for spiritual health, this obedience starts with the physical body, His temple.

If the majority of people are not Christians, we could agree that the majority neither fears God nor believes in divine creation. It follows, then, that most food manufacturers and food regulators do not understand the amazing way that God made our bodies and the ideal food that He provided to fuel them. No limit is present in what can be tampered with in the food supply if there is no fear of God and if the world is believed to be evolving and progressing. Conversely, Christians believe in absolutes that God ordained at the beginning of creation. We can use God-given wisdom to discern how the producing and purchasing of food can please Him.

My purpose is to show the unity between Christian obedience to God and health in our lives *coram deo*—under the face of God. While doing so, I will maintain an orthodox Christian perspective. The Trinitarian God is the Creator and Sustainer of earth and He gives life and breath to all things. God is neither part of the earth (a pantheistic view), nor removes Himself from involvement on earth (a deistic view). God is sovereign above all created things, yet He retains His original interest in His creation and works His will by using the elements of His creation as "second causes."[2] Jesus, the incarnate Word from God, informs our human view of creation, teaching us how to respond to our physical environment. The Holy Spirit renews and transforms our hearts and lives to honor God. As we are renewed, our earthly activities are also directed toward the end of honoring God.

Theology and history are the two disciplines that overarch every area of study and practice. God and His wondrous works are most important for His creatures to know. Understanding the Almighty Creator and King and understanding what He has done on earth across space and time are fundamental to an obedient life *coram deo*. The application of theology and history forms a necessary backdrop to a Christian study of health and nutrition.

Many pagan heresies have surfaced when people evaluate nature by their own sinful reason, and then find a place for a divine being within their understanding of nature. The only proper way to understand the natural world is first to know the God of the Scriptures and His special revelation therein, and then to turn to nature, viewing it exclusively through the lens of biblical wisdom and truth. Going to nature first gives a wrong view of God; going to God first will give a right view of nature.

Praise the LORD from the earth, ye dragons, and all deeps: Fire, and hail; snow, and vapours; stormy wind fulfilling his word: Mountains, and all hills; fruitful trees, and all cedars: Beasts, and all cattle; creeping things, and flying fowl: Kings of the earth, and all people; princes, and all judges of the earth: Both young men, and maidens; old men, and children: Let them praise the name of the LORD: for his name alone is excellent; his glory is above the earth and heaven.

—Psalm 148:7–13

God's magnificent creation, and the reality of sin that alters and conflicts with it, is fundamental to our study of health and nutrition. The rain clouds in the sky, the proximity of the seas, the minerals in the land, the heat from the sun, and the elevation of mountain valleys all have a part in the food that is grown and eaten. The concept of "the one and the many" gives a unified meaning to the discovery of a certain healing herb, to the harvest of root crops on another continent, and to the ripening of fruit in the temperate sunshine, right up to the meal we tasted at breakfast.

People in every culture constantly search for and raise food, making use of the natural things He created and following their created role of subduing the earth. God provides the food we need for different seasons: foods that ripen in the summer are energizing; foods that can be preserved for the winter are warming. God has created a wonderful variety of foods, and God has given man the resourcefulness to use this variety. Mankind was created for God's glory, and creation was established for God's glory. God "satisfieth the desire of every living thing...and preserveth all them that love Him" (Ps. 145:16, 20). Christians should deliberately use what God created toward the praise of His glory.

I sing the mighty power of God, that made the mountains rise,
That spread the flowing seas abroad, and built the lofty skies.
I sing the wisdom that ordained the sun to rule the day;
The moon shines full at His command, and all the stars obey.

I sing the goodness of the Lord, who filled the earth with food,
Who formed the creatures through the Word, and then pronounced them good.
Lord, how Thy wonders are displayed, where'er I turn my eye,
If I survey the ground I tread, or gaze upon the sky.

There's not a plant or flower below, but makes Thy glories known,
And clouds arise, and tempests blow, by order from Thy throne;
While all that borrows life from Thee is ever in Thy care;
And everywhere that man can be, Thou, God art present there.[3]

Is not God gracious? His salvation covenant, His creation for us to live in, His patient teaching when we are slow to learn, His clemency when we fail, His daily provision, His giving us more on earth and in heaven than we could ask or imagine—these realities are all gifts. Any degree of health we have is a gift, because, as sinners, we deserve death. This gift should make us love His commands and seek to please Him—in our lives, families, and future generations.

> O taste and see that the LORD is good: blessed is the man that trusteth in him. O fear the LORD, ye his saints: for there is no want to them that fear him. The young lions do lack, and suffer hunger: but they that seek the LORD shall not want any good thing.
> —Psalm 34:8–10

> "This is the bread which cometh down from heaven, that a man may eat thereof, and not die. I am the living bread which came down from heaven: if any man eat of this bread, he shall live for ever: and the bread that I will give is my flesh, which I will give for the life of the world."
> —John 6:50–51

Mankind is miniscule compared to the size of the earth; one generation is tiny in the epochs of time; humans are like worms compared to our Almighty Creator. Yet look at what a glorious abode God has placed us in—a flourishing planet that sustains us and offers endless opportunities for discovery. Men and women are infinitesimal compared with the rest of God's creation, but have been entrusted with dominion over it.

I thought the following words from a wise Christian doctor aptly contrast God's magnificent glory and the lesser beauty of earth:

> As he spoke, His voice spread through His love and revealed a design that reaches from the minuteness of each single electron to the expanse of the farthest galaxy. Yet in all its brilliance, it was only a dim reflection of the character of the hand that made it. So in the beginning, He created a home, a home filled with light and moisture and rich soils that would be home to the grandest of all His creations.[4]

Then, in the inspired words of the Hebrew psalmist:

> Oh that men would praise the LORD for his goodness, and for his wonderful works to the children of men! Let them exalt him also in the congregation of the people, and praise him in the assembly of the elders. He turneth rivers into a wilderness, and the watersprings into dry ground; A fruitful land into barrenness, for the wickedness of them

that dwell therein. He turneth the wilderness into a standing water, and dry ground into watersprings. And there he maketh the hungry to dwell, that they may prepare a city for habitation; And sow the fields, and plant vineyards, which may yield fruits of increase. He blesseth them also, so that they are multiplied greatly; and suffereth not their cattle to decrease. Again, they are minished and brought low through oppression, affliction, and sorrow. He poureth contempt upon princes, and causeth them to wander in the wilderness, where there is no way. Yet setteth he the poor on high from affliction, and maketh him families like a flock. The righteous shall see it, and rejoice: and all iniquity shall stop her mouth. Whoso is wise, and will observe these things, even they shall understand the lovingkindness of the LORD.

—Psalm 107:31–43

In His world, God created unity: not a unity of things with each other in no relation to God, as New Age belief would propose, but a unity that comes from all things having their origin in one perfect and orderly cause, Jesus Christ. When food is altered and adulterated with processing and artificial chemicals, God's order is destroyed on many fronts. Altered food is not nutritious for the nourishing of our bodily temples. The earth, which we are to steward responsibly, becomes polluted by chemical deposits. Many corporations chase high monetary profits rather than integrity of marketing and the benefit of consumers. I continue to be convinced that problems are not solitary; they are linked to many factors. The way to remedy these problems is to study how we can most please and serve God in every area of life and to study the properties of the things He created, with the Bible as our guide.

In practically every field of study and industry in America today, leaders are getting as far as they can from God's order. Christians need to be aware of this situation and counteract it; if we go along with it, we not only dishonor God but wreak havoc on ourselves. Sometimes, as in secular education, there is a deliberate trend to forsake the God of Christianity and to impede the awareness of the populace. In other areas, such as food processing and regulation, there remains some knowledge of the harm that certain substances bring; yet the same harmful decisions are repeatedly made, furthered by a corporate desire to be lucrative and to grow food bigger and faster. However, the primary cause of food problems occur when people forsake God and the study of His Word and ways; the obvious and unavoidable trend will be destruction and deterioration. Ruining the nourishment that God created for food might not be a deliberate decision, but the desire to preserve nutrients will fade if there is no respect for life and life's Creator and Sustainer.

An understanding that God is Creator of the world and that men and women are the crown of creation will lead to utmost respect of all of God's creatures at the same time as dominion is taken over the animal kingdom. An evolutionary worldview, which perceives men, women, and animals as evolving from the same original type of matter, leads first to exaltation of animals on the same par as humans, and finally to destruction of both animals and mankind. Further insight on this subject is aptly given by Joel Salatin in a recent documentary, *Food Inc.*, where he stated that a culture which views slaughterhouse hogs as inanimate "organisms to be manipulated" can, without much further deduction, start to view certain persons or certain nationalities with "the same disdain, disrespect, and controlling mentality."[5] When I heard that wise and striking statement, I was impressed by the fact that only through an evolutionary worldview do we have an American culture that simultaneously wants to fight against the very butcher of animals and protect exotic endangered species from human contact, yet raise and slaughter hogs for human consumption in the most atrocious way imaginable.

The creationist Christian worldview is the only one which places both humans and animals in their rightful places. This worldview gives mankind the privilege of harnessing the plant and animal kingdoms for the mission of cultivating the earth for God's glory. In a distinctively Christian culture, then, animals will be eaten, yet they are honored for the place they hold in God's creation. Plants are allowed to beautify the earth and fill their place in the ecosystem at the same time as being grown for food. Nature will be channeled and cultivated without being adored, adulterated, or annihilated.

Without a fear of God and His Word, there is no limit to what people and businesses will try to do with the food that they supply to the nation. By leaving godly principles such as truth in advertising and a free market economy, even more damage starts to come as harmful substances become more available and more nutritious things become less available or heavily regulated. (Gratefully, this is not comprehensively the case; Christians can support and even spearhead the growing natural-living sector.) With so many ways *not* to fear God in any area that people set their hands to, what a stimulation this should be for Christians to know the desperate need to fear God in every area of life. While unable to govern the diet or economy of the nation, Christians can govern the diet and economy in their own homes. As more homes obey God in the simple, but profound, things, influence on a larger scale will be more of a possibility.

Christians cannot change a major mode of action and expect everything else in our lives to work well. We cannot eat whatever we want and expect our bodies to stay strong and the earth to stay unpolluted. Searching out how God's world works and how we can cultivate it to please God is a mercy and a blessing. As the Bible, especially the book of Psalms, indicates, God extends untold blessings and mercies to His people when they fear and obey Him. As Christians come to know Scripture, God reveals more to us about His patterns in nature. When we are sanctified, we begin to understand more and more about how to live God's way.

Chapter Two

God Restores the World

"There is not one blade of grass, there is no color in this
world that is not intended to make us rejoice."[1]

—John Calvin

IF "CULTURE IS religion externalized," as Henry Van Til proclaimed, and if diet prefer-ences are an element of culture (which they are, since diet is not universal but is shaped by geography, people groups, and traditions), then all food practices, including harvest, preparation, nutrition, and consumption, are associated with the working outward of a people's religion. Whether a tribe worships the sun and soil, the harvest itself, or the God who gave it, this obeisance is a religious activity. Whether a tribe revels excessively in food and drink or consumes it in disciplined moderation, meals are a cultural and religious activity. A distinctively Christian and reformed view of culture will likewise affect our food preparation and diet choices.

A principle of the Bible, of history, and of this book, is that Christians develop things in an enduring way. While environmentalists are concerned about the preservation of nature amidst "overpopulation," God has said the earth is for man's dwelling and dominion, and for man to cultivate and to exercise stewardship over. God tells Christians to subdue the earth, not to generate substances which abuse the earth's resources. Having stewardship over the earth applies to production as well as consumption. The Christian way to fill the earth is to do so in an understanding way. This means to train children in convictions about stewardship, to obey God by investing in things which will be fruitful and multiplying, and to work in ways which will yield "gold, silver, and precious stones"—works that will last for eternity, works which are the "riches of the nations" described in the book of Revelation.

Yes, spiritual standing comes before cultural work, but our spiritual state is not our only object. Rather, salvation defines and transforms the whole Christian life into one of serving Jesus. Indeed, in God's world, no dichotomy stands between the spiritual realm and physical realm; all things on earth are given by His provision and are to be directed toward His glory. All of our actions will be characterized by the inclinations of either a sanctified heart or by sinful desires. We should study God's will for His chosen people and for the earth, so that our actions are consistent with our standing in Christ and work toward the same purpose on earth that He has worked in our hearts. Developments are good in God's economy, but only the God-honoring ones will be restored in the new heavens and new earth. The good developments of this life are somehow mysteriously manifest in the new heavens and new earth. Possibly, valuable discoveries and accomplishments in the area of nutrition will be given that kind of restoration.

In the new heavens and new earth, we will be given new bodies, but God still cares about our activities on this earth, and the righteousness of these activities. Repeatedly, Scripture speaks of doing our work in obedience to His principles to garner His blessing—doing work for future generations and doing work of significance for eternity. In order for our work to be sustaining *to* our families while on earth and sustained *by* God in the new heavens and new earth, we need to work for the right purposes and with the right principles.

In *Creation Regained*, Albert Wolters explains the future restoration of creation—which he calls a "drama."[2] This teaching of historic reformed theology gives much meaning to the purpose of mankind on earth and for eternity.

> God does not make junk, and we dishonor the Creator if we take a negative view of the work of his hands when he himself takes such a positive view. In fact, so positive a view did he take of what he had created that he refused to scrap it when mankind spoiled it, but determined instead, at the cost of his Son's life, to make it new and good again.[3]

> ...The scope of redemption is as great as that of the fall; it embraces creation as a whole. The root cause of all evil on earth—namely, the sin of the human race—is atoned for and overcome in Christ's death and resurrection, and therefore in principle his redemption also removes all of sin's effects. Wherever there is disruption in the good creation—and that disruption, as we saw, is unrestricted in its scope—there Christ provides the possibility of restoration. If the whole creation is affected by the fall, then the whole creation is also reclaimed in Christ.[4]

As Christians study what God has made, we seek to honor and work within what God has revealed to us about nature in His Word. Non-Christians, however, either leave God's creation untouched (idolizing it from afar), or destroy God's creation (consuming it carelessly.) Christians and Christian nations have historically been the most inventive and scientific. However, the advancements to which Christianity has led can be too easily used for wrong purposes that are destructive rather than enduring.

Transformed by Christ, men and women desire to reflect the good and true beauty He originally created, instead of the sinfully-distorted worldly concept of beauty. Displaying and designing beautiful things is a way to testify of the Lord's creating and transforming power. Demonstrating true beauty in our lifestyles is a way to take dominion over the earth as God commanded; it is a way to bless our families and enhance our homes, showing to others our love for God. Beauty was spoken of in the Bible at creation, in the tabernacle, and regarding people and relationships. True beauty is sought as we cultivate food in the way God created, preparing it purely and wholesomely to nourish and strengthen us, and serving it lovingly at the family meal table. We can use the natural beauty and pleasure of food to build godly culture. Science and inventions not used for God's glory, however, can lead to the making of food products that are not good and wholesome, and which do not beautify our bodies and the earth.

This is my Father's world, and to my listening ears
All nature sings, and round me rings the music of the spheres.
This is my Father's world: I rest me in the thought
Of rocks and trees, of skies and seas;
His hand the wonders wrought.

This is my Father's world, the birds their carols raise,
The morning light, the lily white, declare their Maker's praise.
This is my Father's world: He shines in all that's fair;
In the rustling grass I hear Him pass;
He speaks to me everywhere.

This is my Father's world. O let me ne'er forget
That though the wrong seems oft so strong, God is the ruler yet.
This is my Father's world: the battle is not done:
Jesus Who died shall be satisfied,
And earth and Heav'n be one.[5]

God will make all things new—with no sin or its effects. By God's grace, we still try to keep from sin, though we will be sinless after our bodily resurrection. The issue of our health is similar. Our lives and godly culture require attention on this earth, as God commands, though life will be perfectly restored in heaven.

As Christians, we must not only care about the spiritual health of the heart, but encourage whole-body health by supporting the body with pure and balanced nutrients. There is a God-honoring way to eat just as there is a God-honoring way to behave. To behave well and to eat well are elements of a full-orbed vision for godly life and culture. Indeed, nutrition equips us with the body possible to work for God, as well as defining our view of the earth—our arena for spiritual and cultural actions.

Dr. Paul Jehle tells how the care of our physical bodies is a manifestation of our spirituality. He says that God's nature is manifest in Christian deeds:

> Our bodies were created by God from the dust of the earth (Gen. 2:7) and thus contain all the minerals of the earth in their composition...It is quite obvious that the closer we feed our bodies with the kind of food that agrees with the composition and design of the Creator, the healthier we will be and the holier our bodies will be in their gift back to God.

> Christianity is intensely practical. We cannot simply be content to have Christ dwell in us, without allowing Him to manifest His nature in our works and deeds which involve our bodies. Christians should not be anti-body.[6]

Respected Christian leader Kevin Swanson has explained, "Worship is made up of a recognition of the antithesis (or the difference between the world and the church, the godly and the ungodly, truth and error.)"[7] The perfect, sovereign God is a complete antithesis from sinful, finite, human beings. Who men and women are and how they act is diametrically opposite to who God is and how He works. Worship, for the Christian, is a lifelong activity of honoring God for who He is, a truth we have been brought to see by His grace. Worship, for the Christian, is a lifelong activity of imitating Christ and being conformed to His image as we approach and execute our vocations and lifestyles.

Just like the mortality of God and humanity differs—He is Creator; we are creatures—the way we operate differs. God creates out of nothing, and His results are marvelous and perfect, just like Himself. Man creates out of what God has made, and his results are corrupted by sinfulness and are imperfect. Mankind was told to take dominion both before and after the Fall (see verses in chapter four), so his inventing, building, and designing are good, obedient, and appropriate. However, unregenerate man works for sinful motives, and regenerate man works for God's glory.

Since the whole Christian life is one of worship, our health and nutrition choices need to recognize the antithesis between how our sovereign God works and how sinful man works. Recognizing this principle, Christians are to cast aside the former lusts of our ignorance and be followers of God, as dear children (1 Peter 1:14; Eph. 5:1). Christians need to honor God in producing and consuming the food and other products that are healthy for our bodies to absorb. Food must be grown and eaten in recognition of His ways being higher than our ways, and our ways in need of divine restoration.

> I beseech you therefore, brethren, by the mercies of God, that ye present your bodies a living sacrifice, holy, acceptable unto God, which is your reasonable service. And be not conformed to this world: but be ye transformed by the renewing of your mind, that ye may prove what is that good, and acceptable, and perfect, will of God.
>
> —Romans 12:1–2

God created things whole and pure; sinful man wrongfully adds to or subtracts from them. There are dire consequences given all the way from Genesis to Revelation, if people add to or subtract from His Word. Therefore, God is jealous over the purity and integrity of His Word. I believe He is also jealous over His pristine creation. For example, He expelled Adam and Eve from the Garden of Eden when they failed His commands; He sent a worldwide flood to purge the earth of rampant evil; He scattered the crowds at the Tower of Babel who sought to follow their own purposes in the earth; and finally, He sent His Son, who came to make all things new and restore them for the Father's praise. God's restoration is being accomplished now in the earth, and Christians have the blessed duty of making known, and participating in, the work of our Redeemer and King.

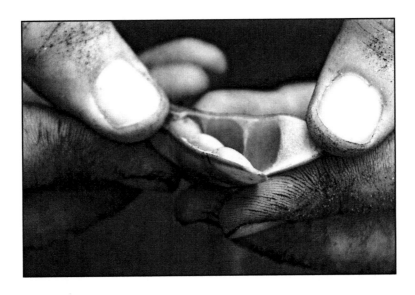

Chapter Three

Wise Physical Stewardship

"If we do not permit the earth to produce beauty and joy,
it will in the end not produce food either."[1]
—Joseph Wood Krutch

GOD OWNS EVERYTHING He created. God is the sovereign disposer of all things.
Our bodies and the earth can be treated as if they are our own, but God has the
ultimate control, and He easily proves it to be so. We must treat our bodies like they are
God's, whose they are. As in salvation when we gave up control of our fleshly will and
ungodly spirit, every area of our lives must yield to the Lord's will. Christians are stewards,
not owners, of their bodies, and are called to serve God, not to work against Him. Each
person is God's living creation, designed to reflect His majestic glory. Our bodies are not,
therefore, vessels to fill with whatsoever the grocery or pharmacy will sell us.

What? know ye not that your body is the temple of the Holy Ghost which is in you,
which ye have of God, and ye are not your own? For ye are bought with a price: therefore
glorify God in your body, and in your spirit, which are God's.
—1 Corinthians 6:19–20

Sadly, there is scarcely a difference between the way that human bodies and the truths
of God's Word are treated by Christians and treated by the world. Little difference is seen
in the outcome of diseases in Christians versus the world, either. For Christians who
profess to have cleansed hearts, who believe that God created all things, and who claim
that God's Word is truth, this record is unfortunate. Our hearts and our bodies are called

unto purity both spiritually and physically. God's people need to live holy, separated lifestyles as part of a testimony to the world and impact upon it.

In order to use physical bodies for God's glory, Christians need to apply wisdom. To do this, we need to seek the purpose for which God created us and the principles He gave us for serving Him. God created mankind to labor and be industrious, to bear and to teach children, and to proclaim His wonderful works among the nations. Strong, healthy bodies and sharp, disciplined minds are instrumental in accomplishing God's plan for us. Nourishing plant and animal life was specially created and suited to sustain us in this important work. Our physical health is an important part of our ability to obey God, though we will never be completely healthy—or completely obedient—until we receive glorified bodies from God.

In their excellent book *Living by Design*, Dr. Ray Strand and Bill Ewing consider health in light of eternity. Again, the emphasized theme is not that health will bring us closer to God, but that godliness will overflow into our health decisions:

> Having a healthy body is not a worthy goal in and of itself. In fact, if we seek that first, we have missed the entire point of our existence. We are called to something infinitely greater and eternally more important: a vibrant relationship with God that overflows into loving service to others and continual worship of Him as our Creator. The body is simply an earthly tool He has loaned us for that purpose. That truth must always come first. Then (if we are wise) we will seek to make that tool efficient and effective as it can be for that purpose.[2]

I appreciate the words chosen by the same authors in the following sentence: instrument, tool, and loudspeaker. These words denote objects that are conduits for greater things—music, a work project, and a message. Indeed, the body does not function as our idol or our destiny; the fleshly body is a channel for the Lord's work.

> ...God created your body to be a vibrant, submissive tool for His work. It is an instrument of praise, a tool for service, and a loudspeaker for truth.[3]

I wonder how the prophet Daniel knew to choose a simpler fare for himself and his friends, and whether he knew the exact physical benefits. Though we are not given that answer in Scripture, Daniel's actions are nevertheless interesting and instructive. Rather than eating the richest, most-select delicacies and wine (prescribed by the king for a period of three years), these young men asked for a plain, wholesome fare of vegetables and water (to be eaten for ten days). Their countenances grew fairer and healthier, and they were noticed for their mental sharpness and unparalleled wisdom. Daniel, in the favor of God, was more knowledgeable about diet than was the king, who thought his prescription would be to the young men's advantage.

And the king spake unto Ashpenaz the master of his eunuchs, that he should bring certain of the children of Israel, and of the king's seed, and of the princes; Children in whom was no blemish, but well favoured, and skilful in all wisdom, and cunning in knowledge, and understanding science, and such as had ability in them to stand in the king's palace, and whom they might teach the learning and the tongue of the Chaldeans. And the king appointed them a daily provision of the king's meat, and of the wine which he drank: so nourishing them three years, that at the end thereof they might stand before the king.

Now among these were of the children of Judah, Daniel, Hananiah, Mishael, and Azariah: Unto whom the prince of the eunuchs gave names: for he gave unto Daniel the name of Belteshazzar; and to Hananiah, of Shadrach; and to Mishael, of Meshach; and to Azariah, of Abednego. But Daniel purposed in his heart that he would not defile himself with the portion of the king's meat, nor with the wine which he drank: therefore he requested of the prince of the eunuchs that he might not defile himself.

Now God had brought Daniel into favour and tender love with the prince of the eunuchs. And the prince of the eunuchs said unto Daniel, "I fear my lord the king, who hath appointed your meat and your drink: for why should he see your faces worse liking than the children which are of your sort? then shall ye make me endanger my head to the king." Then said Daniel to Melzar, whom the prince of the eunuchs had set over Daniel, Hananiah, Mishael, and Azariah, "Prove thy servants, I beseech thee, ten days; and let them give us pulse to eat, and water to drink. Then let our countenances be looked upon before thee, and the countenance of the children that eat of the portion of the king's meat: and as thou seest, deal with thy servants."

So he consented to them in this matter, and proved them ten days. And at the end of ten days their countenances appeared fairer and fatter in flesh than all the children which did eat the portion of the king's meat. Thus Melzar took away the portion of their meat, and the wine that they should drink; and gave them pulse. As for these four children, God gave them knowledge and skill in all learning and wisdom: and Daniel had understanding in all visions and dreams.

Now at the end of the days that the king had said he should bring them in, then the prince of the eunuchs brought them in before Nebuchadnezzar. And the king communed with them; and among them all was found none like Daniel, Hananiah, Mishael, and Azariah: therefore stood they before the king. And in all matters of wisdom and understanding, that the king enquired of them, he found them ten times better than all the magicians and astrologers that were in all his realm.

—Daniel 1:3–20

Christians would not purposefully disable themselves to perform a necessary task; that would be ridiculous. However, we impair ourselves perpetually by eating things which will have detrimental effects on our bodies. Equipping ourselves for performance requires knowledge. Gaining knowledge requires concentrated study when the truth is not readily apparent.

In the following quote, Dr. Joseph Mercola speaks with welcome candor. With these few comments, he calls people back to common sense; with his materials, he reintroduces people to what common sense is. In this way, he is one example of a doctor who is truly a "teacher"—the original Latin etymology of the word "doctor."

> If you take care of your body not only do you prevent disease and illness and prolong your life, but you also vastly improve the quality of your life. You increase your daily energy, creativity, attention span and mental focus, allowing you to achieve more in the pursuit of whatever matters to you...It only takes common sense to understand that what you put in your body several times a day, every day, will have far more impact on your being than anything else you do.[4]

The "common sense" mentioned by Dr. Mercola connotes something that the majority of people have; so why don't most have it? I submit that the decrease of common sense and the rise of degenerative disease today are from a decrease of fearing God and a rise of "every man doing what is right in his own eyes" (Judg. 17:6).

Several things have a lot of impact on us as Christians: the first is our love for God and our mortifying of sin; another is our daily actions as we pursue a lifestyle of honoring Him. Thankfulness to God in prayer is contradictory when we thank Him for the creation of the new day, for our food, for our salvation and sanctification, and then proceed to eat things that contradict biblical principles and harm our bodies. Why pray that we would honor Him with our day if, in the very next thing that we do—eating—we make no effort to find out if it honors His purposes?

The authors of *Living by Design* have diagnosed this trend and expose it quite directly:

> Most of us have asked Him into our lives, but when it comes time for a meal or a snack, we leave Him in the living room as we head to the kitchen.[5]

Caring for our bodies by feeding them what God created goes hand-in-hand with taking good care of nature. Often, food companies carelessly exploit what God created, just to hand the consumer a distorted product—distorted from the way God intended. As Christians, we need to take care of the earth, not because its resources are imagined to be steadily diminishing, but because the Lord commands us to take dominion. Proper dominion honors the sovereign Creator. God created all things well; we need to use the earth wisely and skillfully lest our sin destroy it further.

The first vocations of man involved nature and food. Of course, the natural world was all there was, and food is fundamental to our existence. Adam was the keeper of the garden, and his firstborn son, Cain, was a tiller of the ground. However, they both sinned by using the Lord's gifts in the wrong way and transgressing His commands. God made gardening difficult by cursing the ground and telling Adam that in the sweat of his face would he eat bread. We cannot escape this hardship. In spite of the curse, plants still grow, and men still work and eat. By God's grace, gardening is not harder than it now is, and there remains beauty and enjoyment in growing food and eating it.

We do not use food to serve us (nor allow ourselves to idolize food); we must use food to serve God. Food should not end at pleasing us for our own sake; it should begin and end by serving God's purposes, and nourish us on the way. Since the mind and body are obliged to serve God, food must fit into the same obligation—God's plan, not our own plan. Our plan, carnally, would be momentary pleasure no matter what it costs. God's redemptive plan is for all creation to praise Him and for the generations of His saints to be preserved.

Mankind is still a steward over the ground just like the first man, Adam. Due to sin, however, mankind has the added task of using our bodies as instruments of righteousness. Responsibly tending the earth and conscientiously feeding our appetites are two ways to serve God as stewards of His property. As God cares well for the earth, His people should do likewise.

Thou visitest the earth, and waterest it: thou greatly enrichest it with the river of God, which is full of water: thou preparest them corn, when thou hast so provided for it. Thou waterest the ridges thereof abundantly: thou settlest the furrows thereof: thou makest it soft with showers: thou blessest the springing thereof. Thou crownest the year with thy goodness; and thy paths drop fatness. They drop upon the pastures of the wilderness: and the little hills rejoice on every side. The pastures are clothed with flocks; the valleys also are covered over with corn; they shout for joy, they also sing.

—Psalm 65:9–13

Chapter Four

Laws for the Israelites

"Man shall not live by bread alone, but by every word
that proceedeth out of the mouth of God."

—Matthew 4:4

A S THE DISCIPLE Matthew wrote, man can eternally live only by God's Word. Our mortal lives, even the bread we eat, can be best governed in obedience to the same Word that gives us spiritual light and truth.

God, having created a vast variety of plants and animals, has always been very specific on what was to be eaten. In the first chapter of Genesis, He gave the command for mankind to subdue the earth, including "every living thing that moves," but only plants were permissible for food. After the Fall and the Flood, God repeated His command of replenishing the earth and taking dominion over the animals; this time, He gave a provision for the eating of fleshly meat as well as the "green herb." Animals would begin to eat each other, and humans could eat animals. After God renews the earth, the "lion will lay down with the lamb" once again, and earth will return to a vegetarian society. As long as there is death in the world, though, mankind can kill and eat animals.

And God blessed them, and God said unto them, "Be fruitful, and multiply, and replenish the earth, and subdue it: and have dominion over the fish of the sea, and over the fowl of the air, and over every living thing that moveth upon the earth." And God said, "Behold, I have given you every herb bearing seed, which is upon the face of all the earth, and every tree, in the which is the fruit of a tree yielding seed; to you it shall be for meat. And to every beast of the earth, and to every fowl of the air, and to every thing that creepeth upon the earth, wherein there is life, I have given every green herb for meat:" and it was so.

—Genesis 1:28–30

And God blessed Noah and his sons, and said unto them, "Be fruitful, and multiply, and replenish the earth. And the fear of you and the dread of you shall be upon every beast of the earth, and upon every fowl of the air, upon all that moveth upon the earth, and upon all the fishes of the sea; into your hand are they delivered. Every moving thing that liveth shall be meat for you; even as the green herb have I given you all things. But flesh with the life thereof, which is the blood thereof, shall ye not eat."

—Genesis 9:1–4

The above provision was in place until God gave laws to Israel and specified certain things that would distinguish His people from other nations. A distinction between clean and unclean animals is definitive of the dietary statutes in Leviticus and Deuteronomy. God had promised the Israelites that He would keep them from all the diseases of the Egyptians, and He gave them rules to show how they could obey Him while remaining healthy. The Egyptians did not have the standards for cleanliness of bodies, of meats, or of relationships, such as the standards God commanded that the Israelites follow.

For I am the LORD that bringeth you up out of the land of Egypt, to be your God: ye shall therefore be holy, for I am holy. This is the law of the beasts, and of the fowl, and of every living creature that moveth in the waters, and of every creature that creepeth upon the earth: To make a difference between the unclean and the clean, and between the beast that may be eaten and the beast that may not be eaten.

—Leviticus 11:45–47

In the account of what God provides for His people's food in the first few chapters of Genesis, I was impressed by the fact that there were three-and-a-half times as many clean beasts taken onto the ark, as there were of unclean beasts and fowl. "Of every clean beast thou shalt take to thee by sevens, the male and his female: and of beasts that are not clean by two, the male and his female" (Gen. 7:2). Could it be that, since the clean beasts were to be consumed by mankind, they would be able to multiply more quickly and provide a larger population? Once Noah sacrificed from every clean beast and every clean fowl (Gen. 8:20), there would have been three pairs of clean animals left, and one pair of unclean animals. Whatever the Lord's reason was in commanding this proportioning, it at least shows the importance and the proportional difference bestowed upon the animals that He originally named as clean.

Of beasts that dwell on land, the animals (and their milk) permissible to eat were those that part the hoof, were cloven footed, and chewed the cud. Of creatures that live in the water, the Israelites could eat whatever possesses both fins and scales. Since the type of "clean fowl" was not specified in Leviticus 11 and Deuteronomy 14, the fowl of the air would be understood to be of the same type as the doves and pigeons repeatedly used in the Bible (by Noah in the ark, by the Israelites in sacrifice, and by Jesus at His baptism.) Chicken, turkey, quail, ducks, geese, grouse, partridge, pheasant, doves, pigeons, song birds (and eggs from these birds) would be categorized as clean. In common, these are not birds of prey, they eat insects and plants, they have crops or craws to hold their food, they have three front toes and one hind toe, and they are competent on the ground. Of insects, the locust, beetle, and grasshopper only were clean. All other "creeping things," including other insects, all amphibians, and all reptiles were unclean.

God created the animals and put so obviously into place the distinct differences that mankind has observed in species of birds, fish, and mammals. He used the terms clean and unclean when telling Noah what to bring into the ark, but only at the time of the Israelite nation did He specify what was holy unto Him and what was abominable. Seeing the distinctions between clean and unclean animals is fairly easy. God's distinctions were not arbitrary, but were based on attributes in the animals that He created.

Anything on the land, in the sky, or in the sea that is a predator, a scavenger, or a filter is abominable. These animals eat dead animals (sometimes long-dead), root through human garbage, and soak up pollutants from water, retaining the pollutants in their own bodies. Some of the forbidden creatures were swine, rodents, canines, felines, and equines [horses are not scavengers, but do have parted hooves] of the land; hawks, vultures, and herons of the sky; and mollusks, crustaceans, bottom-feeders, and scale-less fish of the sea. God did not want His people to be defiled by touching or eating these unclean animals. God also told His people not to eat the fat and blood from animals. Many of the unclean animals are naturally quite fatty, giving another reason to avoid them.

In the New Testament, God makes a new covenant with His people that is written, not on tables of stone, but on the tables of sanctified hearts. While He still cares about His people being undefiled (1 Cor. 3:17), spiritual defilement originally comes from the human heart and not from external things (Mark 7:15).

Blotting out the handwriting of ordinances that was against us, which was contrary to us, and took it out of the way, nailing it to his cross; And having spoiled principalities and powers, he made a shew of them openly, triumphing over them in it. Let no man therefore judge you in meat, or in drink, or in respect of an holyday, or of the new moon, or of the sabbath days: Which are a shadow of things to come; but the body is of Christ.... Wherefore if ye be dead with Christ from the rudiments of the world, why, as though living in the world, are ye subject to ordinances, (Touch not; taste not; handle not; Which all are to perish with the using;) after the commandments and doctrines of men? Which things have indeed a shew of wisdom in will worship, and humility, and neglecting of the body: not in any honour to the satisfying of the flesh.

—Colossians 2:14–17; 20–23

For one believeth that he may eat all things: another, who is weak, eateth herbs. Let not him that eateth despise him that eateth not; and let not him which eateth not judge him that eateth: for God hath received him...I know, and am persuaded by the Lord Jesus, that there is nothing unclean of itself: but to him that esteemeth any thing to be unclean, to him it is unclean. But if thy brother be grieved with thy meat, now walkest thou not charitably. Destroy not him with thy meat, for whom Christ died. Let not then your good be evil spoken of: For the kingdom of God is not meat and drink; but righteousness, and peace, and joy in the Holy Ghost.

—Romans 14:2, 3, 14–17

All things are lawful for me, but all things are not expedient: all things are lawful for me, but all things edify not.

—1 Corinthians 10:23

The Apostle Paul shows us over and over again that the kingdom of God does not consist in ordinances, in sacrifices, in feast days, or in meat and drink. These Old Testament laws were temporal and were fulfilled in the person of Jesus Christ. Regarding the themes in these verses, the commentators in the Geneva Bible write that rules, holidays, meat, and drink are not everlasting as is the kingdom of God and therefore are not the priority of our Christian religion. What Christians eat is no longer a command enforced with punishments, as in the days of the Israelite nation. What we eat and when we eat it is no longer a strict, religion-wide practice as it was for the Pharisees and the superstitious Greeks that the Apostles wrote about, or for the Roman Catholics with whom Genevan-era commentators were familiar.

In Acts 10:11–16, God gives a vision to the reluctant Peter, telling him to "rise, kill, and eat" all manner of beasts and birds that were before called unclean. God did not want Peter to break fellowship with the Gentiles over the Jewish dietary laws, but rather to accept those animals as cleansed by God, just as he should accept the Gentiles as able to be cleansed by God (Acts 10:28). It seems prudent that we should not call animals today with the theological term "unclean," since it no longer applies to the Church in the new covenant, regardless of whether we make a conscious decision to eat or not to eat those animals. (When I use the word "unclean" in further discussion, then, I am referring to the Old Testament distinction.)

Taking into account the Scriptures that abrogate the Old Testament ceremonial laws, I have a point to submit. Scientists, and the discoveries that God has given them the insight to make, confirm that the unclean animals that God created are indeed very different from the clean animals. Their digestive systems do not eliminate waste in the same way as clean animals. Their fat harbors the pollutants that are a constant presence in their source of food (garbage and carrion), and their flesh is a breeding ground for parasites. Biblically unclean animals clearly, and detrimentally, affect the bodies of the people who ingest them. "Who can bring a clean thing out of an unclean? Not one" (Job 14:4).

We cannot be sure of the basis on which God separated the clean from the unclean, since we are not told exactly why. Three points deserve mention. God's law does describe the animals based on their physical characteristics such as the chewing of the cud. Swine, one of the most prevalent unclean animals eaten outside of the Jewish nation, is, aside from the law, likened to abomination by the prophet Isaiah. Other Israelite laws, no longer laws to the Church, are yet followed because of health benefits that science has proven, namely circumcision and the washing of clothes and bodies that come in contact with disease. We do not know that God declared animals clean and unclean based on the same reasons that certain scientists have discovered today, but since God is the Creator and the ultimate scientist, I think there is sufficient cause for consideration.

In *Patient, Heal Thyself,* Dr. Jordan Rubin says that, in reference to the Israelite laws regarding unclean flesh, the Old Testament people were "healthier than all of their neighbors" and that "there is wisdom in the Bible that goes far beyond the spiritual."[1] The theocracy of Israel, documented for all time in the Old Testament, was God's special theater for the demonstration of His will and character. Therefore, God's people would do well to give heed to its principles.

One example of scientists discerning a difference between biblically clean and unclean animal flesh was a study done by a university doctor, documented by Dr. Rubin. Animal flesh was added to a growth culture and watched to determine whether the growth was drastically reduced. Scientific observation of God's earth only proves God's Old Testament principles.

> If the flesh substance reduced the culture's growth rate below 75 percent it was considered to be toxic...In all cases, the flesh of the Biblically clean animals was tested nontoxic and the flesh of the unclean toxic.[2]

We use our knowledge and observation to some extent in all of our eating. We do not eat plants which are known to be poisonous to humans. We do not eat a diet of only sugary foods, lest we become sick to our stomachs. The only difference between the things that Christians already know and do, and the actions suggested in this book, is the application of knowledge, forethought, and research.

A principle to be further discussed is that living organisms are influenced by what they intake. Shellfish take in chemicals and harbor them; shellfish were made to do this as part of the ecosystem and food chains that God designed. Since God commanded the Israelites not to eat shellfish, humans are not to be any part of this process in the food chain! If we intake shellfish, we are essentially taking in the harmful properties from which the shellfish have purified the water in which they lived. (With coastal waters continually becoming more polluted with chemical deposits, shellfish from those waters are more toxic than ever before.) If we think about it, God created all creatures and plants and environments to orchestrate amazingly together, providing each other, in the food chain, with all necessary nutrients.

Animals know instinctively what their bodies were made to handle; they are only attracted to that narrow range of foods. God gave people much more variety than He gave animals. Some animals eat only one or two items, but people may eat meat, fish, grains, vegetables, fruits, nuts, seeds, and oils. Is this not enough without grasping for what is biblically unclean or synthetically artificial? Animals eat the way God made them to eat—they do not alter their food. Learning from this aspect of animal life, instead of thinking we should eat all animals, would be very wise. God, while having told man to take dominion, knew that the Israelite diet was of such importance that He filled whole passages with instructions about what to eat of the animals that roamed the earth.

God created animals, and they have not changed. The unclean creatures were unhealthy to consume. Does this matter from the New Testament time forward? Theologically, and lawfully, we may consume the animals that were named "unclean." For health reasons, however, which are possibly the same reasons that God originally outlawed the consumption of unclean animals, we should *not* consume them. While God will not punish us for eating something declared unclean in the Old Testament, nor hold us morally accountable for such decisions, eating them still affects us detrimentally. To the area of our diet, Christians must apply the biblical principles of using wisdom in our lifestyles and being good stewards of our bodies.

Because God designed our bodies, but also gave man the freedom to live in sin, I believe this doctor's statement is true:

> You have the freedom to eat whatever you choose, but when you choose to continually eat things that your body was not designed for, there will be consequences.[3]

Any Bible-submitting Christian that seeks to follow God will end up believing and practicing things which are not specifically commanded. For instance, Scripture tells parents to teach their children the ways of the Lord. Other than using the Bible, we are not told what materials to use to accomplish this; we use godly wisdom as we analyze the options that are available. The same idea applies to our diet. We are to care for our bodies, God's temples. We do all that we can to serve Him, which includes nourishing our bodies so that we are most equipped with the strength and vitality to do His work.

We have liberty in our choice of how we do things. However, we will only retain liberty if we do things in a manner that honors God's design. He made the world and it operates by His laws.

Two American historians expound on this concept of liberty—that obeying God brings the greatest measure of freedom:

> America was built upon the Biblical understanding of liberty. Liberty is not freedom to do whatever we feel like doing, but it is freedom to do what God says we should be doing. God allows men to choose their own paths, but the end of their departing from God's way is death and destruction. Nations that reject God's truth and God's view of liberty will not prosper or advance. The most free nations are those in which individuals and institutions are free to do that which God says they are to do—that is, to perform their jurisdictional functions.[4]

On another note, whoever has invented or installed something is generally qualified to repair it. When operations malfunction in a house, you call a specialist for that system, whether electrical, plumbing, heating, or structural. It is the same with our bodies. God, who designed our bodies and gave them for our use, is the only One who really knows how they work. We need to go to Him for answers when things have gone amiss. Submitting ourselves to the Lordship of Christ means that we are awaiting His leading and His answers to our troubles.

Wisdom, it seems, is knowing enough to understand that we will never know everything and that we must defer to the One who does. Dr. Ben Lerner, who seems to have much knowledge and wisdom about the human body, yet acknowledges that people know nothing in comparison to the intricate, infinite complexity that God created within the human body:

> Because we have no idea what is really going on, all we can do is respect God's ['Body by God'], see its vast potential, appreciate its brilliance, and place no interference in its natural path.[5]

God is ever faithful to hear us and deliver us if we submit to His Lordship and repent of our rebellion. He is abundantly merciful. While biblical promises for deliverance do not guarantee that God will physically heal the earthly life of every person, He does promise to work all things for the good of His people. The promise of deliverance can be understood in terms of God's always protecting His Church as a whole, through the generations. Christians learn from their fathers and mothers in the faith; children learn from their parents. Deliverance operates as new generations seek to follow God more closely than the previous generations did; and God in turn promises to give blessings both spiritual and physical.

> For my thoughts are not your thoughts, neither are your ways my ways, saith the LORD. For as the heavens are higher than the earth, so are my ways higher than your ways, and my thoughts than your thoughts. For as the rain cometh down, and the snow from heaven, and returneth not thither, but watereth the earth, and maketh it bring forth and bud, that it may give seed to the sower, and bread to the eater: So shall my word be that goeth forth out of my mouth: it shall not return unto me void, but it shall accomplish that which I please, and it shall prosper in the thing whereto I sent it. For ye shall go out with joy, and be led forth with peace: the mountains and the hills shall break forth before you into singing, and all the trees of the field shall clap their hands.
>
> —Isaiah 55:8–12

God's people do not know His thoughts, but we can see the general revelation of nature, read the special revelation of Scripture, and learn of His works revealed in history. Nature, Scripture, and history all lead us to a better understanding of God, our Creator and Sustainer, enabling us to serve Him better and live better lives while we do so.

Chapter Five

For Pleasure and Sustenance

"Food is a central activity of mankind and one of the single
most important trademarks of a culture."[1]

—Mark Kurlansky

IN THE BIBLE, food is spoken of in numerous ways in addition to Old Testament laws and New Testament liberty of conscience. One noteworthy theme is that of God providing food for all people regardless of their standing in Christ.

> Sirs, why do ye these things? We also are men of like passions with you, and preach unto you that ye should turn from these vanities unto the living God, which made heaven, and earth, and the sea, and all things that are therein: Who in times past suffered all nations to walk in their own ways. Nevertheless he left not himself without witness, in that he did good, and gave us rain from heaven, and fruitful seasons, filling our hearts with food and gladness.
>
> —Acts 14:15–17

> Behold that which I have seen: it is good and comely for one to eat and to drink, and to enjoy the good of all his labour that he taketh under the sun all the days of his life, which God giveth him: for it is his portion. Every man also to whom God hath given riches and wealth, and hath given him power to eat thereof, and to take his portion, and to rejoice in his labour; this is the gift of God.
>
> —Ecclesiastes 5:18–19

God gives food to all men, by way of the earth, which men have to cultivate and harvest in order to be fed; His Word often speaks of sowing and reaping. The sun, rain, and seasons that He provides to make the growth of food possible are a witness to His life and glory. When mankind labors in the field or labors elsewhere in order to purchase food, meat and drink are his reward and are gifts to take joy in. In Western civilization, where we truly have our portion of "riches and wealth," food can definitely be rejoiced in. Food attentively prepared can give much pleasure—to our eyes as we look upon it, to our taste as we savor it, and to our bodies as it fills us. Certain fruits and vegetables have long been symbols of different virtues and qualities; for instance, pineapple is the symbol of hospitality, and olives are a symbol of prosperity and strength.

Food is something that all people take joy in, one way or another. Whether a child looks forward to his birthday dinner, or a farmer comes from the fields toward the appetizing aroma of a warm repast, or an epicurean tastes the unique qualities of fine cheeses, meals give pleasure. People love to eat what they like—whether they like many types of food, or only select favorites; whether they have their favorites all the time, or only on rare occasions. The cuisines of the world are a fascinating study in the diversity of cultural traditions. Food, after water, is at once the most fundamental need of the human body and one of most celebrated and sophisticated elements of holidays, feasts, festivals, and journeys. Cooking is the limitless art of arranging ingredients, flavors, textures, and colors—an art which many chefs (at home and professionally) have taken to the heights of incredible precision and creativity.

Wonderful meals can bring pleasure to all the senses that God gave us. Food is heard sizzling or simmering on the stove or crunching in our mouths. Our eyes are met by the variety of colors, surfaces, shapes, and sizes that can be manipulated in the process of combining foods and presenting them on the table. Food is felt as it is harvested from a garden, sifted through the hands during preparation, or broken into pieces for eating. Aromas of food often greet entrants of a home even before they make their way to the dining table, and appetizing smells entice us toward what will soon be eaten. Taste, of course, is the one sense dedicated entirely toward food and is the sense, in eating, that is most fundamental. We usually eat only what tastes good to us, though the other senses play a large role in the degree of pleasure we receive from tasting and eating.

Nutrition may be a science, but cooking is truly an art. Meld the two, and you obtain nourishment for all the senses. The following perspective comes from an author from France, a country prized for pursuing the pinnacle of culinary excellence:

> This is why cooking is a real art—like music or painting—that is accessible to everyone and which symbolizes some of the most valuable qualities of life. Perfecting this art should not be limited only to an awareness of the nutritional value of food, but should

also celebrate the culinary pleasures that come from discovering new foods and different ways of preparing them.[2]

The Epistles tell God's people to be "given to hospitality" and "lovers of hospitality." Hospitality means the generous reception of guests; in the way we generally think of it, hospitality includes the sharing of food and the offering of comfortable shelter. In many cultures, to invite someone into your home meant that you would care for all of their needs. To eat with someone meant that you were on peaceable terms with them and would protect them while they were in your home. In the book of James, Christians are taught that the working out of our faith includes caring for the earthly needs of the people that we associate with. Hospitality is not just words, but actions. Whenever the apostles went on their missionary journeys, they stayed in the households of other Christians and shared meals together. Indeed, the last thing that the Lord Jesus Christ did with His disciples was to break bread with them and give them His last instructions.

> If a brother or sister be naked, and destitute of daily food, And one of you say unto them, Depart in peace, be ye warmed and filled; notwithstanding ye give them not those things which are needful to the body; what doth it profit?
>
> —James 2:15–16

Jesus cared for the earthly needs of all around Him while He was on earth. Though God's kingdom is not based on tangible things, but spiritual, we should still follow in the footsteps of how He used common elements to attain His purposes while on earth.

Though food is quite necessary for life and gives pleasure to our senses, a seriousness regarding our diet is crucial. Food is enjoyable, but it should be neither reveled in nor disregarded. I cringe to hear people being careless about their diet. Overweight people who make light of their size; thin people who boast that they eat whatever they want; women who flaunt their fondness for sweets; or men who say they could not care less as long as it tastes good—all of these attitudes show a disappointing levity about a quite serious matter. Ironically, people seem to boast about their addictions to the worst foods. Young people, out of everyone, are most prone to disregard their diet, since they feel healthy and in the prime of life. Notwithstanding the fact that youthful years are the time to invest in good health, health should never be presumed upon.

I have been teased for being interested in health, but I should take that as a compliment. I'd rather have my pantry look like a natural market than a convenience store; like a pioneer's kitchen rather than a chemical-filled factory; and like God's green earth rather than a drugstore. I'd rather be healthy than sickly, and I'd rather be full of God's living food than full of artificial chemicals and additives.

Many people fear that healthy food will not taste good. Actually, it can be very delicious, being made from the wholesome things God created. Whole foods have more depth of real flavor than do artificial and additive-laden foods. Your taste buds will learn to love healthy food, and so will your body as it begins to feel better and give up addictions to chemicals and refined carbohydrates. (Refined carbohydrates and chemical-laden foods *are* addictive, as evidenced by cravings after not eating them for a few hours or days.) Eating healthy for life is not a vogue diet. With healthy eating, you can eat a variety of as many healthful foods as you want without feeling deprived. You will stay fit and trim because healthy foods satisfy instead of causing cravings for more. Healthy food has only benefits—no detriments at all. Food that is all good with little restraint should be something to be passionate about—as opposed to guilt-giving food that is succumbed to then excused away.

I wince to hear people allude to diseases as if they surely will never be confronted with them. Diseases are serious issues, not things to be joked about. I hear people say that one meal of something unhealthy "will not kill me," but this ignorance is quite unbecoming. The truth is that the cumulative use of unhealthful processed food laden with chemicals *is* very harmful. So-called moderation of unhealthy food with healthier food is not the answer; unhealthy food must be avoided.

The "moderate" eating of unhealthy food is *exactly* what large food corporations want you to gravitate toward—and have done much advertising to fool the populace into doing so. Most people know that sugar is not good for them, for example. I wonder whether the same people think that the 120 pounds consumed per capita is a "moderate" amount or an amount lower than it would be if people thought unhealthy food *was* good for them? Regardless, 120 pounds (2.5 lbs. per week) is a large amount.

If you really must eat an unhealthy food on occasion, eat it with knowledge, deference, and thankfulness, but not, please, with bantering or gluttony. God's people are destroyed from lack of knowledge, as Hosea 4:6 tells us. Ignorance about health is not something to make light of, but something to be chased away as soon as possible and replaced with knowledge and understanding.

Sometimes I have heard people mention how bad they know a food is for them, and they eat it anyway. Eating it as the only thing available is one matter, but to eat it in jest is not very becoming to people or to their health. I am reminded of the verse, "Therefore to him that knoweth to do good, and doeth it not, to him it is sin" (James 4:17). Or, as Dr. Don Colbert has said, drawing from his long experience, "most sickness is self-inflicted—either by willful, destructive habits or by ignorance."[3] This is the case, at least, with the illnesses common to Westerners.

Good information is not hard to be exposed to in America. Granted, truth does have a lot of competition, but figuring out what is healthy and what is unhealthy is relatively simple. Americans have so much information at our fingertips, however, that we tend to let it all pass by without letting it affect our self-discipline. Knowledge is futile if it does not bring forth actions.[4] If we continue in ignorance, we will become enslaved to sickness. As Christians, we need to research the truth and apply our knowledge, with wisdom, through our actions.

Since when did epistemologically self-conscious Christians (purposeful evaluators of every subject that influences us) assert carelessness in an issue as vital to us as our diet? The answer is that many Christians have never thought about it, and the same number must think about it.

If we understand sanctification and then health in the proper order, and understand that we should definitely promote the continuation of both, I think two extremes could be alleviated. Indeed, the authors of the following quotation seem to believe similarly, and I was encouraged by the paradigm in their book. They describe two extremes of thought as follows:

> Christians normally show great concern for spiritual growth, yet display tremendous neglect for the physical body. Others are so consumed with physical appearances and health that they have little passion or focus left for eternal purposes.[5]

The answer to why people do not consider their diet is several-fold. One, they feel perfectly healthy. They might feel healthy because God is gracious to give a degree of health even when we make mistakes in our choices. We often have better health than we deserve, given our ignorance. Maybe people think they are healthy because they do not know how much better they would feel and function on a more wholesome diet. Another reason why people do not really think about their diet is because they have taken what is available in stores, assuming it is good for them. Some have heard a claim from one source—such as that milk is good but fattening, and nonfat milk is better—and they never bother with any other research. As long as they eat from the food groups on the most popular USDA food pyramid, people think they have a well-rounded diet.

Our health needs more consideration than we think. Seriously, it does. Chronic diseases, deficiencies, and disorders are at an all-time high. Currently, one in two people will be overcome by heart disease and one in three people will be riddled with cancer. One in two people of minority nationality are projected to acquire diabetes. One in four American children are obese, with this ratio higher (one in three) in non-European nationalities living in America. Cancer has climbed to be the number one childhood disease and number two killer after childhood accidents. Autoimmune diseases, depression, strokes, and digestive diseases are attacking hundreds of people every day.

America has differing health problems from much of the world, and we need to understand their nature before they can be treated. Before giving solutions to the problem at hand, the volume *Nourishing Traditions* sets the problem before readers—a helpful progression:

> Today, chronic illness afflicts nearly half of all Americans and causes three out of four deaths in the United States. Most tragically, these diseases, formerly the purview of the very old, now strike our children and those in the prime of life.[6]

As one doctor has asked, "Why must we accept as normal what we find in a race of sick and weakened human beings?"[7] Do we think the fact of civilization-wide degeneration of health will go away by ignorance? No, it will take vigilance to make a difference in the lives of our families.

Levity and disregard have no place with an issue of such widespread, acute need; neither does apathy have a place in the minds of dedicated Christians seeking to honor God. Not being currently sick is no reason to ignore health. We never know what will happen in the future and should use preventative measures in order to preserve health. In fact, if we continue down the path of the prevalent American diet, there is evidence to indicate that things will not go well with us. At the very least, studying and moving in the right direction is much better than the alternative—disregarding our health.

Before explaining, in her book, how we can locate some toxins in foods, Debra Lynn Dadd explains the foundational and primary purpose of food. While food has many purposes, one is pinpointed here:

> Generally we think of food as something that tastes good, something to socialize over, or something that supplies nutrients, but food plays a vital role in our lives, for the cells and organs of our bodies are literally made from the foods that we eat.[8]

A wise leader and friend, Doug Phillips, has often said that our decisions are made either by default or by design. I submit that whatever your conclusion is after you study health and nutrition, your conclusion needs to be the result of thought and conviction. Will we let people who do not fear God or love His creation decide our diet for us? Many of the people in commercial and bureaucratic entities that determine, regulate, and advertise the food products available are not Christians and do not fear God. Even many Christians do not fear God in the area of health and diet. Will we blindly trust these entities with our dietary decisions?

Please, for the sake of your life, do not go another day without evaluating what you eat and what needs to be changed. Design a set of dietary standards that you will stick to as much as possible. Do not consume anything by default without becoming informed about it and making a deliberate decision to reform.

Richard Baxter, an English Puritan pastor known for his *Christian Directory*, left no subject of practical Christian interest untouched. Below, he focuses on the governing of appetite:

> Understand well what is most conducible to your health; and let that be the ordinary measure of your diet for quantity, and quality, and time...Nature hath given you reason as well as appetite, and reason telleth you, that your health is to be more regarded than your appetite... [Appetite] is irrational, and reason is your ruling faculty, if you are men.

> Poison itself may be as delightful to the appetite as food; and dangerous meats, as those that are most wholesome. So that it is most certain that appetite is not fit to be the measure of a man.

> It is a very great oversight in the education of youth, that they be not taught betimes some common and necessary precepts about diet, acquainting them what tendeth to health and life, and what to sickness, pain, and death; and it were no unprofitable or unnecessary thing, if princes took a course that all their subjects might have some such common needful precepts familiarly known; (as if it were in the books that children first learn to read in, together with the precepts of their moral duty); for it is certain, that men love not death or sickness, and that all men love their health and life...and what an advantage this would be to the commonwealth, you may easily perceive, when you consider what a mass of treasure it would save, besides the lives, and health, and strength, of so many subjects.[9]

Scripture says, "Let your moderation be known unto all men. The Lord is at hand" (Phil. 4:5). Americans seem to overdo everything except discipline in holiness, or self-discipline. We cannot blame large industries for the food they sell us when we have not withstood its temptation. Food purveyors are seeing a market and filling it, but we need not blindly follow. Christians need to make objective decisions. Food industries perceive a wide market, but I see an even larger need for Christians—that of self-discipline and responsible decision-making. Healthy people do not just naturally gravitate toward healthy lifestyles. Any course of action takes decision-making, discipline, and diligence.

A biblical principle that can apply to showing hospitality and to eating food not of our choice is that of authority and submission. God requires that Christians exercise wise rule, under His authority, in the area of personal jurisdiction. In the areas that are not under our jurisdiction, we are to exercise submission to God.

Therefore, in our individual bodies, our families, and our homes, we have the authority to make decisions about the food and other consumables that we buy and use. Even more specifically, parents are in authority over children, and a husband is the head of his wife. Not to exercise authority over the jurisdiction of our bodies and families is to sinfully abdicate the roles that God has ordained. No excuses should be given. If you have a body, and if you have a home, taking charge over it is absolutely essential. Failure to do so is poorly stewarding God's gifts and is falling into laziness where He asks for diligence.

Yet, in some areas we do not have authority. We ought to submit, especially, to the choices of other Christians when in their homes. When traveling, we do not have unlimited capacity to make decisions as we do at home. Choices are limited, and sometimes we find ourselves in a less-than-preferable situation. We can make the best possible choices when we can, such as from a selection of restaurants, but we should trust God and exercise contentment when we do not have that luxury. In restaurants that do not serve according to our preference, we must defer to the circumstances that God has provided and to the hospitality of our hosts—and be thankful. Regarding cases such as this, we should hope, work, and pray toward the conviction that all Christians should honor God in their health and that all people should fear His name.

Hospitality—serving others from your home—is a good opportunity to demonstrate to others the lifestyle choices you have made. Opening your home is an opportunity to make healthy meals and minister to others' wellbeing, nutritiously as well as socially. Just doing what you normally do with healthy food will be an example to people whose diets may not be stellar, and will open opportunities for conversation and sharing wisdom.

Once we can be assured of the fact that we are eating wisely and nourishing our bodies well, food will be enjoyed for more than just the sensory pleasure it gives. After all, true joy and thankfulness should come from our obedience to the Lord, no matter the physical circumstances surrounding us. If we know we are seeking to please God with healthful habits, we will gain more blessing than that of momentary satisfaction.

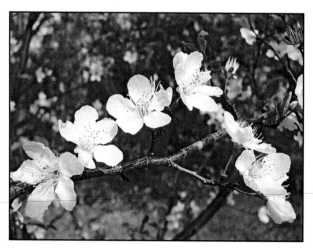

Chapter Six

God's Sovereignty over Health

"Why art thou cast down, O my soul? and why art thou disquieted within me?
hope in God: for I shall yet praise him, who is the
health of my countenance, and my God."

—Psalm 43:5

GOD FORBID THAT, once we have studied and decided upon a more healthful diet, we trust in that for our health. God is the giver and taker of life and health and breath. While we should believe that loving the pure and clean things that He created, and prudently nourishing our bodies with them, will help us to have the best possible health, nothing can guarantee health. Just as the Bible says the wicked prosper for a time, while the righteous struggle under persecution—though God ultimately promises the opposite—there are incongruous cases with health. People that follow all the right principles may have diseases, bewilderingly, come upon them. People that merrily fill themselves with junk food may live far longer than the conscientious consumer. In the end, all people will die, and none will die earlier than the Lord wills it for them.

In my own immediate family, my father died of liver cancer. While it is more assuring to think that his sickness was due to the habits of his younger years, rather than a development in the several years in which we were pursuing a healthier lifestyle, we will never know when his cancer started. I remember, though, that my father enjoyed life and all of God's gifts, was a lover of hospitality, and desired to think biblically about every subject concerning the Christian life. While his death seemed untimely to us, and was a great blow, it is a comfort to know that he was concerned about caring for his earthly body, God's temple.

In God's decree, His saints pass on to heaven and yet God's kingdom continues to advance. This is a mystery to those remaining here below in the arena of earthly service to which God has called us. Those who are left have a greater responsibility to learn from our forefathers and to serve God while we have life and breath.

The unexpected death of my dad is a sobering reminder to the rest of our family. In one way, death reminds us that we should never put our faith in earthly commodities but instead build spiritual treasure in heaven. No matter what Christians do with their bodies on earth, one day they will all be renewed, and God will be no respecter of the persons that comprise His glorious Church. Life is very short compared to eternity with the Lord. Anything that we focus on regarding our earthly bodies must consequently be done for the purpose of serving God. Eternal things are all that matter for the Christian, both on earth and in heaven.

> For he knoweth our frame; he remembereth that we are dust. As for man, his days are as grass: as a flower of the field, so he flourisheth. For the wind passeth over it, and it is gone; and the place thereof shall know it no more. But the mercy of the LORD is from everlasting to everlasting upon them that fear him, and his righteousness unto children's children; To such as keep his covenant, and to those that remember his commandments to do them. The LORD hath prepared his throne in the heavens; and his kingdom ruleth over all. Bless the LORD, ye his angels, that excel in strength, that do his commandments, hearkening unto the voice of his word. Bless ye the LORD, all ye his hosts; ye ministers of his, that do his pleasure. Bless the LORD, all his works in all places of his dominion: bless the LORD, O my soul.
>
> —Psalm 103:14–22

On another note, seeing the terminal sickness of one of our family members is a sobering reminder that we must be careful how we take care of our bodies. My dad became suddenly sick after seeming quite healthy. We will never know on this earth how exactly his disease came about, but that it did is enough to make me hope that we never take disease lightly [see Appendix B for elaboration]. While nothing we can feebly do with nutrition will prevent sickness when God wants to take us home, it is a worthy pursuit to have the most vital lives we can while we are on earth. It is normative to use wisdom to live wholesome lives, and to work for God, not against Him, in advancing His kingdom.

I am humbled by trying to share about health and nutrition, because I have no guarantee of my own health. I certainly do not have all the answers, though I honestly do seek to apply the things I have written. For those that do come down with diseases, nutritional healing is an area of great usefulness, but one that has even more variables and differing methods than the area of nutritional diets. In the following chapters where data is cited, please keep the above caveats and cautions in mind.

Having said that we have no God-given promise of success, I would like to repeat the mission of this book. My purpose has been to encourage the building of godly culture and the designing of mindfully biblical lifestyles. Though we have no guarantee of God rewarding our diligent efforts with good health, one fact concerns us: God does not freely mete out the things that ought to be a result of our own labor. He does not provide endless money; we have to work for it. He usually does not heal supernaturally, but works through the second causes of wise medical practitioners and wholesome nutrition. The Lord is the ultimate giver of all things, but He gives more abundantly to His people who invest in the same ends.

In churches we have visited, it grieves me to hear prayer request upon prayer request for family members or acquaintances that are diagnosed with cancer or tumors or other diseases. Certainly, God's people are right in beseeching Him for their needs, and God is tender and merciful toward His hurting children. Why, however, does the church look exactly like the world in her degree of sickness? God created all we need for staying healthy, barring the sin that prevents us from seeking His will. When I hear prayer requests about diseases, I feel even more burdened that Christians should change their lifestyles before calamities arrive—or else change them simultaneously with praying for healing.

The truth in the first sentence by Dr. Paul Jehle below seems to be held by many Christians. However, he goes on to mention that sickness can also "get our attention," and this is a valuable consideration:

> Sickness, though generally caused by sin, is not always the direct result of individual sins in the life of the believer. Sickness can often be an indicator, a message from the Lord to get our attention so that we seek Him more fully, and in a general sense obey Him more consistently. It can also mean that we simply reap what we sow in that we were poor stewards of our vessels. Thus, to study what makes a body healthy is to study God's design and wisdom.[1]

God is sovereign and can work whatever He wills despite what we think is reasonable or sensible. Yet, in His sovereignty, He has chosen to often work through second causes, that is, work done by mankind.

Hear how the doctrines of God's eternal decree and of His providence are stated in the following excerpts from the Westminster Confession of Faith:

> God from all eternity, did, by the most wise and holy counsel of His own will, freely, and unchangeably ordain whatsoever comes to pass: yet so, as thereby neither is God the author of sin, nor is violence offered to the will of the creatures; nor is the liberty or contingency of second causes taken away, but rather established.[2]

Although, in relation to the foreknowledge and decree of God, the first Cause, all things come to pass immutably, and infallibly; yet, by the same providence, He ordereth them to fall out, according to the nature of second causes, either necessarily, freely, or contingently.[3]

God has commanded that we obey Him and has given general promises that He is the Great Physician, the grantor of long life to those who honor their parents, and the preserver of His saints. God does keep His promises, but not always in the way that we expect. The fact that some Christians die in the prime of life is no reason to disregard His commands, but is rather a reason to hold even more tenaciously to His commands, believing that He requires us to worship Him and trusting that He will work all things well.

Many Christian health resources teach that having peace and resting in what God has done for us is a major component of a healthful body. God is sovereign over our health, and being content with this truth can enhance our health as well. Dr. Ray Strand has said that just as the health of various body parts affect each other, so spiritual health can affect the health of the body, whether negatively or positively, and physical condition can affect the soul.[4] In the book of Proverbs, it is written that "a merry heart maketh a cheerful countenance" and that "a merry heart doeth good like a medicine." (Prov. 15:13; 17:22) The Geneva Bible's version of the latter verse reads "a joyful heart causeth good health." Bitterness, on the other hand, can be detrimental to more than the spirit. As Proverbs 14:30 reads, "A sound heart is the life of the flesh: but envy the rottenness of the bones."

Certainly God has mightily used many men and women who have struggled with chronic illness for their entire lives. They have done God's work in spite of continual physical challenges and have praised God. Suffering men and women, including numerous well-known Christians, have often accomplished more in the midst of sickness than other Christians have accomplished in the midst of health. In fact, we could say that many invalid, struggling preachers, reformers, missionaries, leaders, and hymn writers have spread abroad the knowledge of God and of Christianity in a special way. Their intimate knowledge of hardship and physical pain has allowed them to have a greater grasp on the sweetness of heaven. Their testimonies give us material for studying the merciful works of God in the lives of His saints, and give us reason to consider the history of health and reasons for pursuing it. God uses many secondary and unexpected causes to advance His purposes, yet we must conclude that in general, strong and healthy bodies are very useful for His service. While healthy habits will not prolong the span of our days that God has ordained, they can avert sickness and promote the strength of our lives.

See now that I, even I, am he, and there is no god with me: I kill, and I make alive; I wound, and I heal: neither is there any that can deliver out of my hand.

—Deuteronomy 32:39

O the depth of the riches both of the wisdom and knowledge of God! how unsearchable are his judgments, and his ways past finding out! For who hath known the mind of the Lord? or who hath been his counsellor? Or who hath first given to him, and it shall be recompensed unto him again? For of him, and through him, and to him, are all things: to whom be glory for ever. Amen.

—Romans 11:33–36

Behold, he taketh away, who can hinder him? who will say unto him, What doest thou?

—Job 9:12

Later in this book I go on to compare good, pure foods and poor food products. Some foods, by their nature, will enhance health, while some foods will destroy health. However, as I have said earlier, some people that eat right still get sick and some people that eat junk somehow stay well. What can explain this paradox? I submit that the answer is the sovereignty and glory of God. One of our pastors often says that "there is no *maverick molecule* in this universe"; God controls and commands every single one. Some people seek to honor the principles of God's creation in what they eat, but God can decide to override their health and present them with sickness. Some food is produced, I believe, with no fear of God or respect for His creation, but God can override these motives and use it for His glory in the health of His children. Good and evil, in the end, all accomplish God's purposes. What man intends for evil, God can use for glorious good. What man intends for good, God can use for teaching more humility. Nutrition is not the absolute factor in determining health; God owns that position of determination.

God is not bound by our attempts to be healthy. He can supernaturally bestow health or sickness no matter our decisions. However, *humans* are naturally bound by principles of health. Having a diet consisting of junk food and expecting no harm to come would be foolish. If we conscientiously make wise dietary choices, we can expect a relative degree of health. By God's grace, even food that has been heavily altered by man does have a certain sustaining value; many people are subsisting on it. Yet, if we study the nature of foods, it should be obvious that dangerous additives and processes in man-altered foods *do* slowly deteriorate the body. God allows deterioration to happen in varying measures in different people, but we know for a fact that it does happen.

Unafraid to state what should be obvious, the authors of the next quotation make a correlation with which I readily agree. We often want God to heal us, but don't want to personally promote healing through a disciplined lifestyle.

> The truth is that many of us carry excess weight, do not exercise like we should, and are consuming foods that are far, far from what God designed our bodies to use. Then when our health finally fails, we turn to God for a miracle.[5]

Though He is supernatural and sovereign, God normally works through the natural ways that He made mankind and the whole world to operate. He cares for us in the ways He has promised (shelter and sustenance) by telling mankind to take dominion. Food does not arrive miraculously on our tables, but it does grow for our harvest and further cultivation in fields and forests. God, in His sustaining power, keeps our lungs breathing and our hearts beating, but our research and industry in the fields of agriculture, nutrition, medicine, and homemaking play a large role in the proper care of our bodies.

> Man goeth forth unto his work and to his labour until the evening. O LORD, how manifold are thy works! in wisdom hast thou made them all: the earth is full of thy riches...That thou givest them they gather: thou openest thine hand, they are filled with good. Thou hidest thy face, they are troubled: thou takest away their breath, they die, and return to their dust. Thou sendest forth thy spirit, they are created: and thou renewest the face of the earth. The glory of the LORD shall endure for ever: the LORD shall rejoice in his works.
> —Psalm 104:23–24, 28–31

The choices made toward health not only concern individual lives but have many repercussions in the viability of healthful industries and the lives of our family members extending even to future generations. The fear of God is the unifying factor between knowing that He can mete out whatever afflictions He will, and knowing that we must do our best to care for our bodies, His temples, honorably.

> "The Spirit of the Lord is upon me, because he hath anointed me to preach the gospel to the poor; he hath sent me to heal the brokenhearted, to preach deliverance to the captives, and recovering of sight to the blind, to set at liberty them that are bruised, To preach the acceptable year of the Lord."
> —Luke 4:18–19

Of course, spiritual healing is the glorious and preeminent kind of healing which the Lord gives His children and which we so desperately need. But the presence of something of incomparable importance—salvation—does not omit the need for physical health with which we may better serve God while on earth. Jesus is the only healer and cleanser of our sinful souls. Jesus and His disciples healed many people during their earthly ministry in order to demonstrate God's power and glorify Him. Only He can sustain our lives, and He uses the plants and animals He has created to accomplish the latter purpose.

For bodily exercise profiteth little: but godliness is profitable unto all things, having promise of the life that now is, and of that which is to come.

—1 Timothy 4:8

Although the fig tree shall not blossom, neither shall fruit be in the vines; the labour of the olive shall fail, and the fields shall yield no meat; the flock shall be cut off from the fold, and there shall be no herd in the stalls: Yet I will rejoice in the LORD, I will joy in the God of my salvation.

—Habakkuk 3:17–18

Chapter Seven

Humanism Addressed

Oh, Adam was a gardener, and God who made him sees,
That half a proper gardener's work is done upon his knees,
So when your work is finished, you can wash your hands and pray,
For the Glory of the Garden, that it may not pass away!
And the Glory of the Garden, it shall never pass away![1]

—Rudyard Kipling

SOME PEOPLE CONSIDER care about our health and environment and the desire to use natural products to be "New Age." Such notions are quite uninformed except to the extent that the people who believe those notions are evidently more informed from New Age philosophy than from the Word of God.

First of all, giving up on a significant area of life just because New Age followers have taken a major hold on it is unfortunate defeat. The Bible speaks to every area of life and has the true answers. Christians should apply these answers to their lives and take every thought captive in order to counteract flawed humanistic philosophy with God's victorious truth.

When we look at the steps made in the direction of natural products, many of the steps have been achieved by the ungodly. While we can use non-Christian research and products for our own purposes, Christians should be getting involved in this field and making the advances because God's Word powerfully enlightens our study of health.

I remember seeing a quote on a bottle of Seventh Generation™ detergent and thinking that Christians should be proclaiming such things. It said, "In our every deliberation, we must consider the impact of our decisions on the next seven generations."[2] While I know nothing about the philosophy behind this company—though it does not appear to be New Age at all—I am impressed that the company speaks of human generations rather than just the benefit of the earth.

New Age beliefs are prevalent, however, among many proponents of natural living. "New Age" is a recent term for a philosophy that has been around since the Fall of mankind. Man reveres himself, the creature, and his home, the earth, rather than worshipping the Creator. Any idolatry is essentially humanism, and many forms exist. Some people think man is the ultimate force; some people ascribe the glory to nature instead. New Age philosophy, as it relates to health, could be defined as striving to have our bodies and spirits close to, and in tune with, nature in order to have optimal health and spiritual enrichment.

While striving to have a lifestyle in harmony with the earth, New Age followers can end up focusing inwardly on the unity of their bodies and the earth, leading them to a disposition of worshipping the earth itself as their "mother." As in anything not originating in God, this way of life turns away from God's standard for our bodies to be beautiful temples for Him. Idolatry leads not to comeliness but to doing unsightly things with the body in the name of being natural, and it leads to performing rituals that are not of God.

The Christian's reason for doing anything is methodologically opposed to the world's reasons; even a simple thing such as consumption ought to be an evidence of our redeemed standing with God. Healthfulness will help Christians lead a more useful life, not a more selfish life, because we are not trying to appease the earth but to please our God.

God is the source of all things, not "one" with all things. He gives meaning to all creation. Our quest in following the One True God (who only is real and absolute, unlike New Age pluralism) is to glorify Him. We do not seek to find peace and harmony within ourselves or with an abstract spiritual force, but peace with the Trinitarian God, our Lord and Savior. God is not abstract but has revealed Himself and His will in His Word.

In practice, the Christian's approach to health might fall between modern Western thought and New Age philosophy, but in creed it is distinct from either philosophy. God requires stewardship of what mainstream procedures seem to destroy and what New Age thought seems to venerate—our bodies and the earth. While we should be careful to not poison the earth or our bodies, carefulness is only one of many areas in which to obey God. When we regard our property and our health, we realize that God is the giver, and He created them for Himself. Managing our nutrition is just one component in presenting ourselves as pleasing servants of God.

Humanists try to create heaven on earth and, in doing so, disobey God's principles. Christians know that God will restore the earth and redeem all that is done for His glory, so we seek only to obey God, going no further in our own strength, for we trust in God and know that He will accomplish His plan as He designs.

What numerous authors have said, this selection by Dr. Paul Jehle reiterates. Advice to seek God first, and then His will in various areas of life, is the correct sequence. A correct view of God leads to a proper view of everything else, including health, as it is said so well below:

> The bottom line is the fact that if we begin to make health or exercise, and the condition of our bodies, our god and idol, we will become enamored with self and thus lose the very thing we seek—sound health. One of the best ways to begin a study of the purpose, philosophy, and curriculum of health and bodily exercise is to realize that health and physical fitness begin where all the other disciplines begin, with a correct view of God and His priorities and purposes.[3]

Everything that we do is inescapably religious. We eat either for God's glory or for fleshly pleasure. Will we be righteous or humanistic, serving God or man? Romans 8:5 tells us, "For they that are after the flesh do mind the things of the flesh; but they that are after the Spirit the things of the Spirit."

If we keep our focus on God's creation and provision, our desire to live healthfully will not lead to distorted motives. Then we can live with clean hearts as well as clean bodies. We do not fall into the religions of bowing to the earth or of revering our bodies, nor do we neglect our land, food, and bodies and let them become polluted and impure. The Christian's attitude toward stewardship is a distinct dichotomy from any attitude in secular opinion.

I thought the following quotation, from a university textbook, was rather revealing as to how Christianity can be viewed by unbelievers. I appreciate the evaluation given by these authors, especially in how they acknowledge the presence of worldviews:

> A worldview is reflected in and transmitted through culture. Culturally transmitted beliefs and values shape attitudes toward nature and the environment, which in turn lead to behaviors that can cause or minimize environmental problems...

> The dominant worldview of the United States has been the worldview of the Europeans who colonized North America beginning in the fifteenth century...Christianity, with its roots in Judaism, was a major factor in the development of the Western worldview. Judaism and Christianity proposed a single God who created the universe but was separate from and outside of His creation. A basic Christian belief was that God gave humans

dominion over creation, with the freedom to use the environment as they saw fit. Another important Judeo-Christian belief predicted that God would bring a cataclysmic end to the Earth sometime in the future. One interpretation of this belief is that the Earth is only a temporary way station on the soul's journey to the afterlife. Because these beliefs tended to devalue the natural world, they fostered attitudes and behaviors that had a negative effect on the environment.[4]

I think they are moderately correct about beliefs that are held by Christians; however, I disagree that these are all held by any one Christian. The Christians who believe in cultural dominion are not the same as those who believe that the physical earth is merely a "way station" with little eternal use; these come from different eschatological views and are incompatible with each other. True dominion is stewardship under God, and is not an avenue of exploitation. God will create a new heaven and new earth; hence, our righteous activities on earth are useful for His kingdom and will not be annihilated.

The quotation continues below with a good synopsis of the Industrial Revolution. The authors are quite perceptive in noticing the cause and effect of beliefs on actions, though students of Christian history will likely come to some differing conclusions from those in the second paragraph:

About this time [the eighteenth century, the Enlightenment, and the rise of capitalism] Europe shifted from a largely agrarian or farming society to an industrial one... Consequently, fewer individuals were needed to farm the land. Many people found work in factories, as newly emerging industries developed and flourished... Industrialization brought with it urbanization, as people began to cluster in the areas where the industries were located. People physically separated from daily contact with the land began to lose the knowledge of nature, natural events, and natural phenomena—a knowledge that can best be called a sense of the earth—that had been handed down through generations...

The dominant Western worldview, with its emphasis on the exploitation of nature and resources, the accumulation of wealth, faith in science and technology and belief in the inherent rights of the individual, was a powerful and aggressive force. The Europeans who migrated to the New World found a wild and beautiful land of seemingly unlimited natural resources, peopled by natives who had a far different worldview. For over three centuries, the descendants of these settlers enjoyed the confluence of a large resource base, the technological means to maximize use of this base, and the social acceptance of maximum use of resources. The result was what has been called the frontier mentality, a mindset that encourages the aggressive exploitation of nature.[4]

I thought this passage was quite insightful about the impression Christians can give to unbelievers based on the very ways we use and treat the natural environment. The generationally-transmitted "sense of the earth" mentioned in the passage *has* undeniably been diminished to the same extent that post-Christian America has forsaken her victorious theology and Protestant work ethic. People are watching what we do: will we treat the earth as the careless of the world do when we are claiming to have a noble, holy purpose to our lives? Will we show less care for God's creation than environmentalists who, even in their evolutionary mindset, are being careful of their actions?

The Western worldview, birthed in the Reformation and carried to America by the English Puritans and Scotch-Irish, did not begin with the above intent of "devaluing the natural world." American settlement began with the fear of God and the desire to follow the wisdom of Scripture alone in the earthly advancement of His kingdom. The Spanish, backed by the Holy Roman Emperor, may have settled South America for "the accumulation of wealth" and the "exploitation of nature," but the British settling North America generally had a different view. Families, backed by their pastor and investors in the old country, were intent on forming permanent colonies for the propagation of the Gospel. Attempting to be peaceable with the natives, early Americans formed a society based on responsible property ownership, the free-market development and trade of resources, and God's Word as the only foundation for true liberty.[5]

Protestant Christianity developed the best things in Western Civilization, especially in America, which was Christian from her inception. Today the only thing wrong with the advances gained from those foundations is the absence of the fear of God. In agreement with the quotation, men do now use their relative liberty to exploit the environment, and they put their "faith in science and technology" as the above authors wrote. Christians need to show the nations, once again, the proper way of using God's resources. We need to apply our theology to our lifestyles so that we are not seen by humanists as "devaluing" the natural world and as living schizophrenic to our profession of faith. We need to teach our children to love God's creation, His Word, and His works in history, so that our children will carry on the generational mission of living on God's earth, His way, without being viewed as exploiters of the earth. However, we answer ultimately to God. Humanists that serve man will always have negative impressions about the actions of Christians serving the Lord.

Chapter Eight

Biblical Principles Applied

"To preserve health is a moral and religious duty, for health is the basis of all social virtues. We can no longer be useful when we are not well."[1]

—Samuel Johnson

INHERENT TO THE way God created us to learn and grow are several principles. Biblical principles are evident in the way we are sanctified and transformed, in the way we study and classify the world around us, and in the way we gain knowledge and act upon it. There are two main principles to be addressed which apply specifically to food and to our bodies, and after explaining them here, I trust they will remain obvious in the issues later discussed.

- *Internal before External*
- *Parts to the Whole*

"Internal before external" means that the internal composition of something is manifest in its external characteristics, and the external is a true indicator of what is internal. "Parts to the whole" means that the whole is the sum of its parts, and to get the desired whole, the parts must be in their proper place. The exterior of anything, or the whole entity, is worth nothing more than—and nothing aside from—its interior value and its individual parts.

The spiritual state of our lives is reflected in our beliefs and actions, the internal affecting and finally transforming the external. It is a biblical principle that our souls must be saved and our hearts arrested by God's truth before we will begin to love the deeds of righteousness more than the deeds of sinfulness. Reforms that are forced upon one's behavior will have no lasting impact unless the heart is convicted and the soul is saved by God. Hence, the best way to teach children is first to show them that such-and-such statements are true and then that God calls them to obey Him through obedience to their parents. Setting down rules or boundaries without showing why the rules are right and necessary is the humanistic or moralistic way to teach and is doomed to failure.

The influence of internal matter on external matter is much the same process in our physical bodies as it is spiritually. What we intake leads to what we are and how healthy we are. If we eat improper foods, our organs will not be functioning optimally, and malfunction and deficiencies will eventually be noticed in our external appearance—in our countenance, posture, hair, skin, teeth, and weight. The internal mental discipline of declining unhealthy foods will affect and change an external propensity to hand such foods into our mouths.

Even more fundamentally, what goes into food affects the food's healthfulness for us. Pesticides sprayed on maturing produce are retained in the end product that reaches supermarket shelves, and traces of pesticides are now found in human blood, ultimately compromising our health. Cattle fed on high-starch corn and grain become fatter more quickly than if they were fed on grass. The unhealthy fattiness of the beef that results is determined by what the cattle have taken in. People eating grain-fed beef more easily convert it to excess bodily fat than they would if they ate grass-fed beef. The plant or animal's exterior is the result of what it becomes from the inside outward. People, consuming plants and animals, repeat the same process: taking things in, and becoming characterized by them.

Many parts and many elements contribute to our whole being. The Bible speaks of many virtues and fruits of the Spirit that are important for a Christian life. The epistles to the New Testament churches are full of lists of duties for hospitality, for eldership, for marriage, for churches, and even for the civil state. If a part is missing, the whole will lack that same element. Parts compose the spiritual maturity and mental intelligence of the whole person. God does not merely command us to be complete and good Christians. He gives the details of how to do this—in every area of life. Desiring the whole result without achieving the steps and various parts is futile. Trying to do things in a "whole" way without explaining the parts is the humanistic way. Trying to administer a "whole" concept all at once is not an influential way to teach; this style of teaching does not teach anyone to evaluate an issue, as no understanding of the various parts is encouraged.

In our bodies, the various input received always contributes to the health of the whole. We need a proper diet, adequate rest, and vigorous exercise as the components of a healthy body. Even more fundamentally, our organs require specific nutrients. Organs function individually but are interrelated; each part must be nourished in order to support health in the whole.

In the foods we eat, we must be knowledgeable about the components of the end product. The end product is what we end up eating, but many processes have been involved before that point—processes that either increase the quality and quantity of nutrients, or diminish them. Bread is not just bread! The "parts" of bread might include whether the wheat is whole grain or refined, whether fiber is present, whether the sugar is raw or processed, whether preservatives or flavorings are present, and who you are supporting with your purchase. Each part having to do with the ingredients of bread has an impact on our bodies. Any food that has been manufactured in any way contains parts that affect the whole. Every food that we put into our bodies affects our whole body, since we cannot manufacture nutrients except from the food that we eat.

As in people's character, where many things are not immediately visible on the outside, food is identical. Something taken in, whether wicked images or unhealthy food, might seem harmless until it manifests itself later after taking root in the mind or in the diet. The fact is, Christians are so desensitized to what purity and goodness are, whether in our character or in our health, that we do not know what blessedness we are missing.

Another example about external appearance, coming from a slightly different angle, could be the Pharisees of Jesus' time. To other men, the Pharisees *appeared* holy and pure because they gave attention to their public behavior. But God, who looks on the heart, saw uncleanness and iniquity. God admonished the Pharisees to cleanse first what was within, that the outside would be clean also.

> Woe unto you, scribes and Pharisees, hypocrites! for ye make clean the outside of the cup and of the platter, but within they are full of extortion and excess. Thou blind Pharisee, cleanse first that which is within the cup and platter, that the outside of them may be clean also. Woe unto you, scribes and Pharisees, hypocrites! for ye are like unto whited sepulchres, which indeed appear beautiful outward, but are within full of dead men's bones, and of all uncleanness. Even so ye also outwardly appear righteous unto men, but within ye are full of hypocrisy and iniquity.
>
> —Matthew 23:25–28

On the surface, our body and our food may look similar to the next person and their meal, but what has been ingested by plants and animals and eventually our bodies makes all the difference. For instance, culinary oils can all look the same to the eye's perception, but they can have very extreme effects on the body. Dr. Bruce Fife has said that "oils are masters of deception. You can't tell a rogue from a saint." He writes that toxic oils appear just as pure as freshly-extracted oils.[2] Indeed, oils all look similarly thick, translucent, and yellow-colored to the eye unless we know their molecular structure and their history—the parts that make up the whole.

The knowledge about the process that any oil has undergone is what makes the difference in whether we eat it. Two different oils can have drastically different effects on the body—one for good and one for ill. Though the oils may look the same as each other to begin with, their "parts" are not the same and the "whole" of the human body will become more and more like the kinds of oils eaten—whether toxic or pure, as in the above citation.

Fruit and vegetables can have similarly deceptive appearances. The general public desires unblemished, outwardly perfect food in every season of the year.[3] Pesticides and herbicides are used to achieve blemish-free food, yet those sprays are harbored in the fruit or vegetable, destroying vitamin content and eventually accumulating in the human body. Organically-grown or garden-fresh produce *can* look just as nice, but the results are not consistent enough for most growers and most buyers. Perfect shapes and sizes of produce come with a cost—the interior pollution that will likewise contaminate its consumer.

A truth of the Christian life is that we should not always have what our carnal flesh desires. Since fleshly desires often stem from carnal motivations, desires should be thoughtfully and spiritually evaluated before we give in to them. As the Holy Spirit sanctifies our hearts and renews our mind, our bodies can be disciplined to follow the dictates of a conscience that is becoming godlier. We first need to be instructed in God's principles, then exercise self-denial and obedience as we follow those principles—even in the area of health. We must put to death the lust of the flesh—such as addictive food. Our physical bodies will become, in reality, cleaner and purer as they intake healthy food as a direct result of our mind and spirit becoming more sanctified through godly wisdom and personal discipline.

> The internal state of man's heart is the general cause of his external state individually and culturally.[4]

After the above statement, the treatment of health and fitness in Dr. Paul Jehle's curriculum *Go Ye Therefore...and Teach All Nations* continues on, giving insight on how to apply biblical principles to the teaching of health and contrasting those principles with humanistic methods. He teaches that while Christianity promotes accountability in a life of stewardship, humanism seeks momentary pleasure regardless of the consequences. A Christian view of nutrition seeks to get to the root of the problem, but a humanistic view of medicine would try to cover up the problem. For Christians, the ideal we strive for is to trust in God's sovereignty for our health and eat for His glory; but the humanist's ideal is trying to eat the way toward good health, for human satisfaction.[5]

There really is, therefore, a way to glorify God with our eating habits versus glorifying self. The eating habits of a culture really are shaped by the attitudes and religious beliefs of the people. Each of the comparisons that Dr. Jehle made shows that Christians have distinctive methodologies that should be played out in our lives. Our eating habits *do* reflect our worldview, so we had better make certain that we are starting with a careful Christian worldview. If we do, our view of nutrition will parallel Dr. Jehle's remarks: we will seek accountability and stewardship, and we will seek to get to the root of problems. We will eat for God's glory if we start with the premise that God must be glorified in all things.

Another principle to consider is that "bad company corrupts good morals." Bad things contaminate good things and pollute purity. You may have a nice herbal tea, but if you add artificial sweetener into it, it changes from a beneficial tonic into an injurious liquid. You may have organic chicken breasts, but if you cook them in the microwave (to be further discussed in chapter fifteen), the nature of the poultry is changed for the worse as newly-formed free radicals vie for influence in your body. You may have whole-wheat toast, but if you spread margarine on it, any good elements of the bread are overcome. Just as one drop of color taints an entire jug of water, one artificial or chemical substance alters the food's intended impact on your body.

Foods of inherent goodness have few, if any, caveats attached to them. The quality of food tends to take care of the quantity. It is easy to overindulge in processed, sugary foods because sugar causes cravings for more sugar, but people typically do not eat an excess of spinach or brown rice; these are good for you, but not addicting. The nutrients that are helpful for one ailment are helpful for another because they are inherently, wholesomely, *good*. For instance, whole grains help to keep blood sugar lower for people caring for their diabetes or obesity; whole grains also supply vitamins and fiber to prevent cancer and aid in digestion. However, the foods that are unwholesome—such as refined white flour—contribute to and may result in any number of maladies; they clog the intestines, create free-radicals in the body, attack the immune system, supply "empty calories" devoid of vitamins or fiber, raise blood sugar, and lead to increased hunger and therefore overeating.[6]

I hope you will keep those principles in mind as you continue reading. Points I make and suggestions I give are only the "tip of the iceberg," though I trust they will be consistent with my theme and will encourage your own thoughts and research. Much beneficial material exists—and seeks to lead people into a healthier lifestyle. As we all begin to understand how the internal brings about the external and how parts make up a whole, there are a few additional items to remember while forming a system of beliefs and practices.

Do our choices respect wise principles?

- A regard for divine creation and the natural world?
- A regard for the diet and laws of biblical times?
- A regard for our national history?
- A regard for present scientific evidence?
- A regard for future generations?

Do our decisions show prudence in the following areas?

- An understanding of each element that can be analyzed within a finished food product.
- An understanding that everything that goes into food production affects its final composition.
- An understanding that the integrity of what we take in directly influences what we are on the outside.

If a diet or trend radically compromises any of these areas, if it seeks to change the external apart from the internal, or if it seeks to address the whole instead of its parts, then that diet is likely unwise to follow. May we study the Scriptures with a mind toward God's will for our health, and then approach our lifestyle choices with a determination to let godly wisdom transform our lifestyles from the inside, outward.

In the following declaration, Dr. Ray Strand and Bill Ewing have what I think is a visionary perspective. Eternal principles can be lived out here and now, and our lives can be preparation for eternity. We live our lives not in a totally separate realm from eternity, but as the journey toward eternity.

> This is one of the great rewards of living by design: to take eternal principles and begin to apply them now—so that the feast, the parade, and the celebrations might begin now.[7]

I consulted the aforementioned principles to evaluate the research material I used, judging the material by the principles since I am neither a scientist nor a nutritionist doing original exploration. If you agree with the principles outlined above, I hope that you will be open to seeing current nutritional wisdom encapsulated for you in subsequent chapters and to seeing biblical principles applied to its analysis.

Chapter Nine

A Culture of Endurance

"Thus saith the LORD, Stand ye in the ways, and see, and ask for the old paths, where is the good way, and walk therein, and ye shall find rest for your souls."

—Jeremiah 6:16

TAKING A THOUGHTFUL look at the culture around us, it seems obvious that instant gratification is the description of almost every activity. From church messages that give sound-bites of sentiment, to drive-through fast food, to rapid transportation and internet connections, our culture seems to be collectively impatient. Impersonal automation is clad with the worthy-sounding names of efficiency and productivity. Capitalism and swift advancement in technology induces a desire to have the latest in electronics, entertainment, science, and comfort—and not only the latest, but as many options as possible. There were 870 different items in a grocery store in 1928, four thousand in 1952, and eight thousand by the 1960's.[1] Today, there are 47,000 different items clamoring for recognition on store shelves.[2] (Despite this "illusion of diversity," as Eric Schlosser stated on his *Food, Inc.* documentary, there are "only a few companies involved" and "only a few crops involved."[3] After all, that's the easiest way to make food manufacturing happen faster and more cheaply.)

Will America ever be content without continual exponentiation of mechanized processes or selection of goods? Will America ever be content without continual fractionation of the time that it takes to accomplish a given task—whether raising a steer to maturity or eating it for dinner at a drive-through?

While progress is an avenue of man's dominion taking over time and resources, progress can become so consuming that we do not realize our reliance on it. The areas of food and health are especially affected by the paradigms of popular culture. The main point of modern advertising seems to be selling food that is the quickest, easiest, tastiest, and makes the consumer the happiest. With people's busy schedules, those attributes are understandably appealing. Quickly-prepared foods are usually processed or packaged foods; easily-eaten foods are usually refined and preserved, needing little preparation; tasty foods are usually loaded with the unhealthy fats, sugars, and flavors that people have become accustomed to in convenient foods. Promised satisfaction is determined by how much you want the food, not whether you should have it.

Actually, the advertising of food is an interesting concept; advertising never had to be done two hundred years ago. I wonder, what would we be eating if we did not have television, flyers, billboards, and coupons? Wholesome food hardly needs advertising; God displays it for us on His verdant, fruitful earth. But then, in secular thought, modern man is thought to have progressed beyond the ways of our ancestors. What is progress, therefore, and how should we analyze it?

One area of progress, modern healthcare, is phenomenal in its ability to protect life, to handle medical emergencies, to diagnose diseases, and to perform complex surgeries. This is a valuable, ancient field of work and a great accomplishment of mankind. However, we should not put explicit trust in allopathic healthcare, and should exercise a few cautions. External care cannot replace internal sustenance. Most healthcare professionals believe that nutrition has little, if anything, to do with curing diseases. Typical doctors and nurses are well-meaning, of course, and are noble in their efforts, but are following the only thing they have been taught. Allopathic (mainstream medical) practitioners will usually prescribe drugs before thinking about preventative or natural curative measures. Most drugs help in one area but harm in many other areas.

Though the latest medical developments and discoveries are astounding, much of latest medical theory is heavily influenced by the same ideas that plague all of popular culture: the belief in quick fixes or cover-ups of the real issue, and the belief that the most prevalent opinions on health are valid. As far as surgical operations and life support, the work of doctors and scientists is more than admirable. However, when it comes to treating symptoms of disease with synthetic pharmaceuticals, rather than using natural methods or exercising prevention beforehand, conventional medical philosophy is flawed and even corrupt at times.[4]

Another area of progress is technology—an outworking of man's God-given dominion ability and a discipline of much benefit to society. Often, however, Western philosophy funnels its focus on technology and forgets to give regard to the natural landscape, our contact with it, and use of it. Material in the earth provides all the resources for technology, but once we have the technology in place, we tend to forget about the source. God created the natural world to be beautiful in itself, not just as a place to be trampled in the pursuit of man's concept of beauty. Dr. Jordan Rubin warns that in our forward technological progress, we must not become disconnected from nature. "It is in our best interest to maintain contact with the good earth," he states.[5]

I have noticed that in old books, beauty is described as coming from a strong, well-formed figure and a bright countenance, usually due to health. Today, however, modern advertising assumes that beauty comes from adorning the outside of the body. Beauty can only come from the outside, I suppose, when nutrition is not beautifying us from the inside to the outside. Letting ourselves decay on the inside and then covering up the decay from the outside sounds too similar to sin, such as lying and then lying more to protect oneself. A healthy diet, rather, leads to strong nails, shiny hair, and glowing skin—the very things that are often covered with various colors and finishes because they are pale and brittle otherwise.

Dr. Weston Price has studied the bodily structures and teeth of small, isolated people groups all over the world. The teeth in tribes whose diets are untouched by Western civilization are beautiful, shapely, healthy, and strong, as a result of good nutrition. This doctor's work is like a glimpse into history—a glimpse of people groups untouched either by import of the Western diet or by emigration to Westernized countries. Today, Americans need replacements, coatings, and fillings in order to improve their dental appearance. Our diets are not maintaining health and strength for us. Without inferring that necessary dental work or some enhancement from makeup is wrong, I deem that cosmetic work that makes us into something far different honors neither God nor our bodies. Dental and cosmetic work often imitate the condition we would be in if we had sought a healthy lifestyle. Should we not follow God's ways so that we may reflect His beauty with shining countenances and bodies fit to work?

The trends of popular culture (were we to adhere to the extreme that secular advertising offers) lead to unhealthiness, obesity, and disease. Popular culture, however, praises and celebrates the very opposite. The covers of magazines in grocery stores showcase slender and pretty models, yet inside the magazines are found advertisements for factory-grown chicken, corn syrup, drugs, and refined foods—all of which bring real disaster into the body.

In the spiritual realm, temptation and sin promise you one thing and leave you with an altogether different result. Many magazines and advertisements do the equivalent by promising that which popular culture worships (youth, health, beauty, and ease) but delivering the poor consequences of a lifestyle saturated with popular culture (disease, skin-deep looks, and futility.) What appears right in man's eyes is wrong in God's sight.

While many advances of Western Civilization (in the sciences, education, commerce, cleanliness, lifespan, reduction of plagues, and standard of living) are in large part due to the Christian religion and the fear of God, recent health practices are definitely not an advance. Indeed, entrepreneurship and capitalism have expanded the variety and availability of food, and charitable associations have been able to spread our abundance to poorer countries. Increase is accomplished. Unfortunately, the American brand of "nutrition" is being exported all over the world, lending a crutch to countries with little supply and production. Monetary poverty has no relation to health among people who supply their own food, but poverty does have a relation to health when people groups become reliant on food that is bestowed and do not have the knowledge or finances to eat better.

As in anything that begins with godly principles (civil freedom, for example), freedom may become abused when people cease fearing God. Freedom has been glorious for America, but when freedom is taken for granted and not preserved by God-fearing leaders, freedom becomes useless. Such is the case with health. In this country, we have the technology to import food from worldwide, we have a wide selection of food in practically every community, and we have the money to pay for these choices. For people without the fear of God, desire is the dominating consumption factor and greed is the dominating production factor. The actions or foods that make most people immediately richer or happier are the ultimate goal. The heritage of prosperity that we have as Americans will do no good unless we continue to fear and serve God.

America's food crops have not, at this point, suffered from famine, plague, or pestilence—the difficulties with which many countries of the world are attacked from without. Rather, America is attacked from within by an unseemly reliance on the riches available; we have too much culinary abundance and too little discernment. The message for American health, then, will be different from a message to less-Westernized parts of the world. America is not stricken by deficiency of resources; she is stricken by laziness and carelessness amid wealth of resources. "For unto whomsoever much is given," reads Luke 12:48, "of him shall be much required."

> God told the Israelites, "For when I shall have brought them into the land which I sware unto their fathers, that floweth with milk and honey; and they shall have eaten and filled themselves, and waxen fat; then will they turn unto other gods, and serve them, and provoke me, and break my covenant."
>
> —Deuteronomy 31:20

Food is manipulated in every possible way, and Americans think it is all progress—yet the populace is wasting away. We are stricken by poverty of knowledge and ignorance of history, not by poverty of food. We are so self-confident that we will fall headlong into disaster if we do not look back to reference history and the rock-solid foundational truth of Scripture. When nations and cultures stop fearing God, they degenerate—no matter how technologically "advanced" the nation is. When our food choices do not acknowledge God, our bodies degenerate—no matter how technologically "advanced" the food is. Nations and cultures operating in the fear of God have historically made the best and truest advances.

Dr. Paul Jehle of Plymouth Rock Foundation writes of our American heritage of health as it came from the Reformation in Europe. I appreciate his linkage of the Bible as foundational and this foundation leading to the protection of freedom and then the advancement of health.

> [The Reformation] opened up God's revelation in all areas, including health. Europe became a leader in stemming the great plagues and diseases through obedience to the laws of God. This was because it had received the Bible into its culture...

> The Constitution of the United States provided great freedom medically and most practice was private and successful. Due to the free enterprise atmosphere, many inventions and progress was [sic] made in the medical field...

> The prosperity and health of America were testimonies to the obedience of her people to the basic laws found in the Bible. Each individual was responsible for his own health plan, and also responsible for its consequences.[6]

Since all of Scripture is useful for correction and instruction, I think the following passage written to the people of Israel is particularly applicable. America is a nation likewise birthed by an abundant measure of God's providence and yet, in enjoyment of these blessings generations later, she is in danger of forgetting God as the source of her prosperity. The next verses are God's serious warning to the Israelites.

> For the LORD thy God bringeth thee into a good land, a land of brooks of water, of fountains and depths that spring out of valleys and hills; A land of wheat, and barley, and vines, and fig trees, and pomegranates; a land of oil olive, and honey; A land wherein thou shalt eat bread without scarceness, thou shalt not lack any thing in it; a land whose stones are iron, and out of whose hills thou mayest dig brass.

> When thou hast eaten and art full, then thou shalt bless the LORD thy God for the good land which he hath given thee. Beware that thou forget not the LORD thy God, in not keeping his commandments, and his judgments, and his statutes, which I command

61

thee this day: Lest when thou hast eaten and art full, and hast built goodly houses, and dwelt therein; And when thy herds and thy flocks multiply, and thy silver and thy gold is multiplied, and all that thou hast is multiplied; Then thine heart be lifted up, and thou forget the LORD thy God, which brought thee forth out of the land of Egypt, from the house of bondage; Who led thee through that great and terrible wilderness, wherein were fiery serpents, and scorpions, and drought, where there was no water; who brought thee forth water out of the rock of flint; Who fed thee in the wilderness with manna, which thy fathers knew not, that he might humble thee, and that he might prove thee, to do thee good at thy latter end; And thou say in thine heart, My power and the might of mine hand hath gotten me this wealth.

But thou shalt remember the LORD thy God: for it is he that giveth thee power to get wealth, that he may establish his covenant which he sware unto thy fathers, as it is this day. And it shall be, if thou do at all forget the LORD thy God, and walk after other gods, and serve them, and worship them, I testify against you this day that ye shall surely perish. As the nations which the LORD destroyeth before your face, so shall ye perish; because ye would not be obedient unto the voice of the LORD your God.

—Deuteronomy 8:7–20

As Christians, we need to be concerned with integrity and endurance, not wealth, popularity, or novelty. We need to be informed about durable things. In health, integrity consists in foods that the Bible speaks of and which are proven to be healthy. Honestly, I have a hard time accepting that recently-held beliefs are going to counteract the recent rise in diseases. One such belief is that some natural foods (pure butter, coconut oil, etc.), long-eaten in the past, are harmful for human consumption. Healthcare is one of the largest industries in Western Civilization—the same culture that has almost entirely left the dietary practices of our ancestors! American diets have radically changed, necessitating unprecedented advances in medical research. The technology surrounding the processing and marketing of new-fangled foods, and the medical inquiries attempting to make sense of nationwide epidemics, are both costing billions of dollars which were historically unnecessary.

At the beginning of her whole foods cookbook, the following author traces how Westerners had for more than a century gotten away from knowing the healing power of food and again are becoming interested in this science:

Throughout history, every culture has used food to prevent and treat illness and disease, and promote good health...However, around the time of the industrial revolution, people in Western countries came to disregard the medicinal and therapeutic properties of food, and it is only relatively recently that interest in the healing qualities of food has been revived.

This renewed interest, owing to our growing concern about what we eat and drink, and our quest for good health, is spurred on by scientists who have undertaken extensive research into eating habits, and have also investigated the properties of individual foods.[7]

Which substances were not present in the diets of our healthier ancestors? Refined sugar and high fructose corn syrup, enriched white flour, hydrogenated oil, pasteurization, preservatives, additives, synthetic flavorings, artificial colors, and poisonous chemicals. Processed carbohydrates, processed meats, processed fats, and processed foods of every combination. Things that come only in packages. Things that have too little life to even decay. Things that have nutritionally-bankrupt calories. As they have been commercialized, foods have lost the dietary value of enzymes, vitamins, minerals, fiber, phytonutrients, and good bacteria.

The advent of the twentieth century brought, to name a few things, the manufacture of flaked cereals, the growing prevalence of commercial bakeries, the invention of hamburgers, the introduction of iceberg lettuce, the United States' first pizzeria, the sale of Coca-Cola™ in every state, and the marketing of canned foods.[8] Around the time of World War II, America saw the founding of McDonalds™ and Dairy Queen™; the marketing of sugarless sweeteners and cake mixes; nearly half of the agricultural workforce leaving farms (moving from eighteen percent of the workforce in 1940 to ten percent still on the farm in 1960); the number of bakery workers increase to thirty times the number of fifty years previous; and the use of preservatives such as BHA.[9] The number of food inventions and convenience products has only increased during the last 120 years, much to the chagrin of our health and home life.

Families of the past must have enjoyed living closer to the natural environment than most Americans do today. Families kept themselves supplied with clean wilderness meat and fish, juicy fruit from orchards, crunchy garden vegetables, and fresh whole grain bread. Glass jugs of raw milk, pies cooling on the windowsill, and herbs hanging in the cellar conjure a striking image of yesteryear. Agrarian lifestyles, though involving intense labor, exposed people to the harmonious simplicity of God's creation. It would have been normative to eat foods as whole and as fresh as it is possible for food to be.

Whole foods are not appealing because they are old-fashioned, however; they are appealing because they are *timeless*. Good food endures, not in the sense that artificial preservation causes endurance, but in the sense that good food will always nourish and sustain life—whether in our great-grandparents' day or our own or our grandchildren's day. Search, therefore, for the food that is timelessly appealing and timelessly nourishing.

Though we should regard the history of foods and of eating, I do not mean to indicate that the health of people in the past was ever without hardship. Certainly, there have been food shortages from weather and war, awful plagues that wiped out entire cities, and prevalent diseases due to unfortunate diets. We are blessed today to be less concerned about famine and epidemics. However, due to Western prosperity and knowledge, the kinds of diseases that are rampant today are almost pathetic. We have never had more of the world at our disposal than we do today, yet we take little thought of how we employ our resources.

Though always learning from our ancestors, we do not wish to return to the era in which they lived. We want to glean all possible wisdom from them for infusing to our own generation. Even further, we want to pass down wisdom to be perpetuated with our descendants. Commenting on Solomon's ancient inquiry, "Say not thou, What is the cause that the former days were better than these?" (Eccl. 7:10), the English Puritan Matthew Henry wrote the following:

> It is folly to cry up the goodness of former times, so as to derogate from the mercy of God to us in our own times; as if God had been unjust and unkind to us in casting our lot in an iron age, compared with the golden ages that went before us...God has always been good, and man always bad; and if, in some respects, the times are now worse than they have been, perhaps in other respects they are better.[10]

In countless ways, technology makes our lives easier. Technology is hardly worthy of its name, though, if it does not improve upon something. Irresponsible technology is not laudable. Progress must be combined with wisdom if progress is to have integrity and longevity. Here we find true ingenuity and dominion—in the application of wisdom to keep in check the advances of technology. In any area of learning and education, progress is not chasing whatever is happening; progress means to be continually learning, evaluating, and modifying. Improvement comes by using the best ideas and principles as a foundation for forging new ground and scaling new heights. Our pursuit of health in what we eat and manufacture must be the same way.

Insofar as it makes food more accessible, technology is most profitable. Insofar as it renders food more unhealthful, technology's true profitability for society is diminished. For just as the food industry knows about artificially preserving food, the American people have lost their knowledge about naturally preserving food to retain the nutrients and eat it before it spoils. Refrigeration was not in use one hundred years ago, and people had to use other methods of preservation—such as drying, canning, and fermenting. In my opinion, the greatest achievements in the last twenty years have not been technological, but have been from people noticing the adverse results of American diet trends and striving to counteract these trends with excellent practices.

Albeit in his guide to improving education, Kevin Swanson of Generations with Vision has a helpful analysis of technology. Not everything can be made more efficient, he believes. Indeed, efficiency is not the only commodity to be pursued. There are other worthwhile things such as relationships and simplicity:

> In many ways, technology has fooled us into thinking that everything now is new and improved. We thought the industrial revolution would make everything more efficient. In the end, there were some things that could not be made more efficient: the relationship developed and the lessons learned by a son as he plowed the fields side by side with his father under the hot summer sun; the time spent on the front porch between grandmother and granddaughter as they snapped the beans and peeled the apples; or the long winter nights shared by a family in close quarters, playing the fiddle, reading out loud by candlelight, and maybe even telling a tall tale or two. With all our technology, division of labor, and efficiency, we have come to discover that we cannot manufacture relationships as we do everything else. There are some things you simply cannot delegate. There are some things you cannot make more efficient by mass production. There are some things you cannot automate. It will always be that way.[11]

"There were some things that could not be made more efficient," Mr. Swanson writes regarding relationships. Another thing related to technology which cannot be made more efficient, I submit, is nutrition. Quality food requires time, space, and attention to grow, prepare, and eat—else its quality necessarily diminishes. Additionally, automating the production of food eliminates many good *relationships* such as the symbiosis, or mutual benefit, between animals and plants. Another relationship could be the harvesting of your own garden alongside your children and the intangible satisfaction that comes from the process. Food quality that is dependent on slow, natural processes cannot be reached to the same extent if food is mass-produced. For instance, naturally fermented cucumber pickles used to be a trove of nutrition, but since the advent of commercial canneries, we are left with a similar taste but none of the good bacterial properties of fermented vegetables. With increased efficiency, traditional quality declines.

Technology used in growing large quantities of food and importing and exporting it all over the world is commendable. However, when the advances of technology start to exploit natural food by refining and processing, technology has no true benefit. Manufacturing that began several centuries ago as human ingenuity for the purpose of better supplying food and serving mankind has gotten out of control. Food processing today stops at no limits of quantity and continually sacrifices quality on the altar of profit. Factories in and of themselves are not faulty; my only concern is that factories tend to be used for refining and changing plant and animal foods to a far greater extent than home cooks or small companies with limited machinery could ever do.

We need not let technology govern us, however; we can use what we need for our advantage to the extent possible without letting it harm us. We must exercise the capability to make our own decisions and not take every food that is offered. American abundance blinds us into thinking that we need it all—and fast. Let us instead look at this abundance from a godlier perspective by thanking Him for His provision, and admiring the ingenuity of people, but considering the health of His temples before greedily accepting what is the most abundantly produced or easily acquired.

The buy-now and pay-later mindset seems to be prevalent everywhere in popular culture. Enjoy sin now and deal with the consequences later. Get into debt and enjoy luxury now so you (or your children) can worry about it later. Expend your health while you are young and deal with the repercussions later. Fill your mind or body with junk (images, noise, food, or drugs) with no thought for what the results will be as it accumulates in your system. Thinking only of the moment and of human satisfaction is not a trait of Christianity. God would have us to remember His works, invest in the future, and glorify Him through His creation and through our minds and bodies. We can, by God's grace, make responsible use of the many wonders of the world—the environment created by God as well as technology developed by man.

A keen analyst of history, Doug Phillips of Vision Forum Ministries has pronounced the following warning gleaned from the history of civilizations:

> The most astute and technologically diverse and advanced people will be destroyed, not from without, but because of the morality crisis from within.[12]

The Western food industry is technologically advanced. America knows how to modify genes, to develop crops resistant to herbicides, and to separate plant matter such as wheat kernels into every possible component. We hydrogenate oil and homogenize milk (processes both invented at the start of the twentieth century) and practice many other methods of producing and processing, fractioning and refining. While mankind has always been technologically advanced to an extent, the modern industrialism, particularly that of food production, is unprecedented. Man's precise technological advancements are indeed quite scientific and stretch the very limits of discoveries. Mostly, however, science is pursued completely without God and will therefore tend toward destruction. Scientific pursuit must be built on a premise of fearing God in order for it to accomplish truly great and enduring achievements.

Knowledge or power will not save us; faith and the fear of God will save us. All the advances in the world will do nothing to preserve our civilization if we idolize food or wealth or convenience or youthfulness rather than submitting to God, worshipping Him, and obeying His precepts. Westerners have decided to operate our own way (i.e. as in diet), and have then begun to trust in our abilities—and we are reaping the consequences of this crisis.

If they lack a solid foundation of God's truth, actions and philosophies will collapse like houses built on sand. God is not fooled by external "progress" when internal spirits are rebellious and decaying. We must honor Him with reverent hearts and build any technology upon this foundation lest the technology destroy us. The Bible says it is "the righteous [that] shall inherit the land, and dwell therein forever" (Ps. 37:29).

Here is an example of the food industry tampering with what God has created. Coconuts and their oil were particularly provided by God for the people of tropical regions. The properties of coconut oil are well-suited to the needs of those people, since the oil protects against sun damage and an environment filled with harmful insects and plants. According to some observers, the people of the Pacific Islands are some of the most well-proportioned and beautiful people in the world. Coconut oil has been an integral part of their diet and an instrument of their good health for thousands of years. Pacific Island women typically had large families of fine, healthy children.

The following research by Dr. Bruce Fife is in a similar vein to that of Dr. Weston Price's aforementioned research of traditional cultures. It is a shame that the islanders, in many instances, changed their traditional diets while probably trusting the processed Western foods offered to them. The islanders had their long-standing culinary traditions, but their traditions, presumably not based upon conviction, were easily traded for modern products. (The same thing happened in twentieth-century America.)

> Coconuts have been a staple in the diets of Pacific Islanders for thousands of years...But until their adoption of modern foods, heart disease and other degenerative conditions were unheard of. Heart disease only appeared in island populations after traditional foods consisting of coconuts and coconut oil were replaced by modern processed foods and refined vegetable oils.

> The early explorers who visited the South Sea islands in the sixteenth and seventeenth centuries described the islanders as being exceedingly strong, vigorously built, beautiful in body, and kindly disposed. The islanders gained a reputation for their beauty, excellent physical development, and good health...Such observations may have even fueled interest in the folklore of a fountain of youth.[13]

Tropical oils (coconut and palm), because of their stability and resistance to rancidity, were once used for frying foods. In the last one hundred years, however, these oils have been replaced by the newfangled procedure of hydrogenation of unsaturated vegetable oils. The U.S. government-subsidized soybean industry has overwhelmed the commercial food industry and deceived thousands of people by claiming that soybean oil is better for the heart than the "unhealthy" saturated coconut oil.[14] Heart disease has skyrocketed to its current place as the second-highest killer in the United States. We should be very careful about using a new product until its results are proven—desiring rather to stick with food that is traditional and demonstrated to be healthy.

The problem with employing new products and concepts is that they have no history and therefore come with no guarantee that the products will do in the future what they are thought to accomplish now. While we often tend to think that eating something one time will not hurt or help us; this idea is false. Everything affects our bodies, especially with continued use. Endurance, instead of present momentary pleasure, must be carefully considered. Years of healthy eating will fortify the body and build the immune system; years of unhealthy eating will become revealed in problems that can take years to counteract.

New things have different possible philosophies attached to them and are not bad in themselves. In salvation, Christ renews our sinful natures and transforms us to "walk in newness of life." He grants new perspectives and new desires. However, we need to know about the past in order to remember God's work in history and His sanctification of our past sinful habits. Humanism, on the other hand, favors new things in order to get away from the past and cares only for progress (if from an evolutionary mindset) or a standstill (if from a fatalistic mindset), caring neither about sin nor purity. As we seek new discoveries in health, or new lifestyles and nutritious diets, we need to be rooted in the past and what it teaches us.

When something new is brought on the scene, especially in the food industry, we have no understanding of its effects. The safest course of action is going back to the old paths wherein our forefathers and mothers walked. A Christian principle is to hold fast to what we are taught and assured of without swaying toward contradictory advice. While the following verses are speaking of Bible doctrine and do not directly refer to health, I submit the belief that the Bible does inform our view on health and we should heed its inspired words as truth straight from God our Creator.

> But continue thou in the things which thou hast learned and hast been assured of, knowing of whom thou hast learned them; And that from a child thou hast known the holy scriptures, which are able to make thee wise unto salvation through faith which is in Christ Jesus. All scripture is given by inspiration of God, and is profitable for doctrine, for reproof, for correction, for instruction in righteousness: That the man of God may be perfect, thoroughly furnished unto all good works.
>
> —2 Timothy 3:14–17

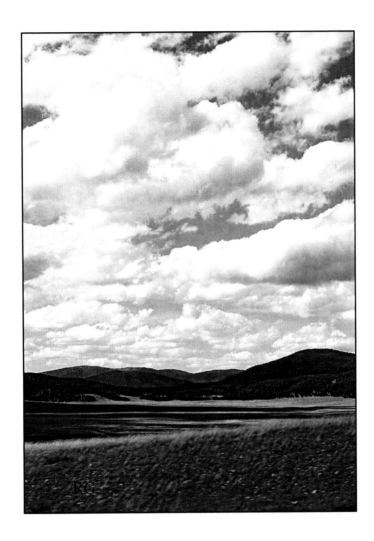

Chapter Ten

Toward Multiple Generations

"Liberty is to the collective body, what health is to every individual body. Without health no pleasure can be tasted by man; without liberty, no happiness can be enjoyed by society."[1]

—Thomas Jefferson

BIBLICALLY-MINDED CHRISTIANS SHOULD be interested in the works of the Lord in history and in the advancement of God's kingdom in the future. Historical events and future events have a bearing not only on our spiritual walk, but also on our physical lifestyle, including nutrition. By learning of the practices of our ancestors, we can understand how they remained healthy. By nurturing our own health, we can invest in the health of our children and their children. Christians should learn from the past in order to use the present in preparing for the future. The ways of our ancestors presently teach us—and our generation was once the *future* progeny for whom we would have wanted our ancestors to prepare. The Holy Scriptures tell us to "Remove not the ancient landmark, which thy fathers have set" (Prov. 22:28). Endless wisdom may be gleaned from referencing the past.

The history of food is fascinating. We can research food availability in certain places at certain times and the diseases that people struggled with based upon the diet they consumed. We can learn how foods were typically prepared. With capitalism and commercialism aiding in easy acquisition of food, many homemakers have never learned about using natural remedies and have never learned about preserving food. Food-as-medicine or food-preservation can be studied, but we will not learn it as thoroughly as if it were

71

passed down from our great-grandmothers. Many people speak about their grandmother's prolific gardening or cooking as a lost art that the next generation did not follow. This discontinuity is unfortunate, yet traditions can be revived. It may take a few years to learn the things we were not taught while growing up, but it can be done.

The book *Nourishing Traditions* speaks of our forebears' ingenuity in preserving food and aiding digestion by the fermentation, soaking, and sprouting of milk, grains, and vegetables. In earlier times, people did what they could with locally obtainable foods and tools. They skillfully used herbs to treat infirmities. None of our billion-dollar healthcare facilities existed, but people knew so much more than we do about nature. Our early American and European ancestors were more closely connected to their food and observed how it affected them, but we tend to be removed from our food and know next to nothing about it. God has provided everything we need to live; we ought to search it out. Technology is a blessing in many ways (for instance, we can take herb capsules rather than growing the herbs ourselves). Technology, however, is not necessarily the best development ever seen by the world.

After World War II, natural—organic—agricultural practice became the alternative method rather than the norm it had been historically. The new norm became what we now know as conventional agriculture, which is characterized by industrialized genetics, farming and processing, and by chemical pesticides, herbicides, hormones, and additives. World War II was also the unprecedented occasion of women starting to work away from their homes. By doing so at the same time that industrialism increased, women were not as attuned to traditional methods of food preparation nor to the needs and the health conditions of their families. Roughly seventy years later, we can reflect on the country's position: The majority of women work outside the home, lamenting their lack of homemaking and cooking skills whenever they are at home. Often hand-in-hand with this career trend is a culture of fragmented families and fast-food subsistence which, it can be argued, are major factors in the drastic decline of health in Western nations. The sake of health is one reason why women should manage their homes and know the needs of their families; this is a great work, yet on a different front than men's work.

More sharp insight by Dr. Jehle on our American history follows. Notice his mention of the government's actions since World War II, as well as his suggestion of what must be restored—individual responsibility for family health. Both of these concepts are helpful here but will be a key foundation to the discussion in chapter fifteen.

As the centralization of American life took place in the economic and civil spheres, so it did in the medical field as well. Slowly but surely the health and welfare of individuals became a collectivist responsibility of the federal and state governments...Persecution through regulation of homegrown natural foods and new inventive solutions to harmful diseases, under the guise of safety, has been the pattern of government agencies since the Second World War...We need to restore a respect for human life, and also a respect for the inventive talents of individuals to take responsibility for the health and welfare of their own families.[2]

The lifestyle developments in the last seventy years are a prime illustration that Christians should be extremely careful before falling for the newest trends. Where will these trends lead in fifty or sixty more years? Are they leading in the right direction? History is a precious teacher. Unfortunate consequences come when people do not fear God, for He is in control and His promises for blessing and cursing are steadfast. Following God brings blessing even on our health, such as when women will manage their homes and take time to "give meat to their households" (Prov. 31:15)—an action God esteems to be virtuous. Going astray always brings damage. Americans did not foresee that chemical agriculture would pollute the land and seas and wreak havoc on our health, or that children's health would decline with mothers absent in the work force, but God knew. God set principles in place ranging from the stewardship of the earth to the stewardship of our homes. It does not go well for the wayward. A long-term vision is necessary to counteract the trends which have been so long in place (at least since World War II.) But we must, must, must be faithful! God multiplies blessings to those who "keep His commandments to do them," in ways we cannot know or imagine.

For Christian families who desire to have children trained in godliness, and to have this legacy continue for many generations, health should be a primary facet of study. Why?—because health is passed down. People are more likely to contract a disease if it was existent in a family member. Healthful habits are easily lost if they are not taught to the next generation—which is exactly why we are no longer following the good practices of our ancestors. Conversely, we can invest in the health of our progeny. The health of the pregnant mother, before and during pregnancy and nursing, has a large bearing on the health of the child—on the mother's carrying to full term and on the child's skeletal structure, immune system, brain development, and overall health. Common knowledge indicates that caffeine, alcohol, and tobacco smoke can harm the unborn child. Wholesome high-fat and high-protein foods will proactively benefit the unborn child. The facial formation of the sinuses, nostrils, jaw, and dental arch is understood to be very much related to the health of the parents. The condition of both sets of teeth (juvenile and secondary) is much affected by the prenatal health and early diets of children.

The health of the child in his youth will set the stage for his health during the rest of his life. To give an example of a child's delicate needs for a pure environment, the author of *The Organic Food Guide* claims that "up to 35 percent of lifetime exposure to some carcinogenic pesticides occurs by age five."[3] The youthful years are the time of the most growth and the time most in need of the best nutrients. Youth is the time to train children's appetites toward wholesome foods and exercise carefulness over the things they eat or are offered to eat. A child's food preferences are formed in the first few years of his life, starting in the mother's womb. Children will probably gravitate toward unhealthy, sugary foods if such are available. During the early years, the mother should especially control the intake of her children and ensure a wholesome diet. Much research suggests that the diets of children have an enormous impact on not only their strength and immune systems, but also on their mental capacity and behavior. Undernourishment, usually caused by disproportional sugar and refined carbohydrates, can contribute to hyperactivity, lethargy, aggressive behavior, and depression. Children's minds and bodies should be as best-equipped as possible in order to serve the Lord.

Unlike the world, where parents make decisions and hope their children make good decisions too, Christian parents want to train their children in what they know is right, which is following God wholeheartedly in all things and faithfully keeping God's covenant. Parents should want to teach their covenant children every aspect of their Christian lifestyle (as commanded in Deuteronomy 6). Our diet and health decisions form a major foundation for our lifestyle.

Food and harvest are directly related to God's generational blessings upon His people, and this very theme is to be taught to children, as is seen in the following passage.

"And it shall come to pass, if ye shall hearken diligently unto my commandments which I command you this day, to love the LORD your God, and to serve him with all your heart and with all your soul, That I will give you the rain of your land in his due season, the first rain and the latter rain, that thou mayest gather in thy corn, and thy wine, and thine oil. And I will send grass in thy fields for thy cattle, that thou mayest eat and be full. Take heed to yourselves, that your heart be not deceived, and ye turn aside, and serve other gods, and worship them; And then the LORD'S wrath be kindled against you, and he shut up the heaven, that there be no rain, and that the land yield not her fruit; and lest ye perish quickly from off the good land which the LORD giveth you.

"Therefore shall ye lay up these my words in your heart and in your soul, and bind them for a sign upon your hand, that they may be as frontlets between your eyes. And ye shall teach them your children, speaking of them when thou sittest in thine house, and when thou walkest by the way, when thou liest down, and when thou risest up. And thou shalt write them upon the door posts of thine house, and upon thy gates: That your days may be multiplied, and the days of your children, in the land which the LORD sware unto your fathers to give them, as the days of heaven upon the earth."

—Deuteronomy 11:13–21

Parents instinctively try to keep their toddlers from things with potential harm, such as eating bugs or dirt, playing with trash, or touching surfaces that harbor germs. However, these same parents will intentionally give their children foods that are equally harmful—if not more harmful than germs and dirt since food's effects are subtle. With only a little attention it would become obvious that refined sugars and carbohydrates, artificial additives, sodas, and candy not only inhibit proper childhood growth but also begin to produce damaging effects.

In his fabulous book *Body by God*, Dr. Ben Lerner tells of the normal American way he was raised, shows how detrimental this "normal" was in his own life, and appoints a better plan. Dr. Lerner says that his favorite childhood foods were all made of dairy products, sugar, chemicals, unhealthy fats, and refined carbohydrates. A litany of infections had him continually visiting the doctor, and misbehavior had him continually visiting the school principal. However, as Dr. Lerner writes, not one person connected his diet with his health or his behavior.

I appreciate the way he explains that bodies of children are essentially *created* by what they eat as they grow and develop. This is so fundamental, but often forgotten. While nutrition for an adult functions mainly as maintenance and repair, nutrition for a child functions as the foundation and building materials.

> Unfortunately, although I was continuously ill, my nose was always running, and I constantly struggled to keep quiet in a classroom, no one ever considered the possibility that my problems may have been related to all the sugar, dairy products, caffeine, and food coloring coursing through my veins.

> The proper feeding of a child is incredibly important as their ['Body by God'] is completely being created by what they are eating. Sadly enough, the tendency is for children to eat more junk, refined foods, and sugars than adults. This disrupts God's intent for their once perfect little bodies and has a deleterious effect on their future.[4]

Since Christians normally believe in diligently training their children, behavior is usually attributed to discipline—the practice of it or the dearth of it. Proper training in righteousness is biblical (Eph. 6:4). However, parents need to obey more than the command to discipline children rightly; parents need to *nurture* their children with the good food that God created. Children are *provoked* to misbehavior when they are sustained on sugary and blood-sugar-raising foods while they are being instructed to calm down, pay attention, and obey.

As Christians, we attribute violent behavior to wicked hearts. Rebelling against God in any way *is* wickedness, whether in relational behavior or in destroying His creation.

The use of God's creation and the manifestation of human conduct are not separate: Diet has been found to make a difference in behavior. The scarcity of B vitamins (whole grains and legumes) and good oils (non-hydrogenated oils and unaltered saturated fats), and the profusion of refined carbohydrates, artificial sweeteners, and chemical-stimulant beverages have been documented to generate disruption of the body's systems and to promote extreme mental and nervous behavioral conditions. The most obvious reason responsible for this imbalance in standard American diets is an unhealthy proportion of omega-6 fatty acids to omega-3 fatty acids. Omega-3 fatty acids are fundamental to mental and nervous system health.

Poor diets contribute to low intellectual capacity and deficient mental function; there is a remarkable correlation between crime and delinquency and inferior mental constitutions.[5] Could it be that the far-from-nutritious Standard American Diet and the escalating crime rates go hand in hand? Could sin in one area, leaving God's design for our personal diets, be leading to sin in another area, more crimes committed against persons and property? The fact is well established that a healthful lifestyle contributes to a positive, cheerful attitude and a superior level of purpose and energy—the very opposites of the characteristics of criminals. Parents need to give special attention to their children's physical growth as well as their spiritual training; without either provision, as is the case in many worldly families, more children will become liabilities in their communities.

While teenage rebellion should not be excused, I wonder if junk food diets have anything to do with their behavior. Nutrition is vital in the developing adolescent years and will set the stage for their health as mature men and women. While many homes do not have stellar health practices to begin with, the odds for eating nutritiously are lessened if teenagers spend most of their time away from home and readily subsist on a diet of junk food. The truth that diet affects our behavior should be an area of close attention as it regards the solid growth and well-being of Christian children.

It has been reported that if juvenile obesity continues to increase at the rate it currently is, today's generation of parents may *outlive* their children. The worst foods are marketed to children, and many children, left at the mercy of popular culture's standards, alternate between daycare, school, and other institutions, having no consistent caretaker of their health.

Mothers especially need to invest in their own health before carrying children, need to eat nutritiously while they are nursing, and need to feed their children nutritiously all through their youth. If this standard is set, and children are trained to desire wholesome food, they should desire to continue a healthy lifestyle their whole life and raise their own children the same way. Basically, whole families need to eat healthfully all of the time! Some people groups have practiced special diets for women before marriage and childbearing because they understood the importance of the mother's health in raising the next generation of hearty boys and girls for the continuation of their society.[6]

A person's health is not isolated if they are part of a family. Surely, the choices we make affect those around us, particularly our descendants. Would we intentionally cause them to be unhealthy? May our most basic action, eating and drinking, equip us for our most essential action—worshipping God in and with our lives.

Chapter Eleven

Meals for Family Culture

"When a woman stays at home and cooks with good judgment and understanding, peace and happiness result. She thus controls the family's health and destiny, also her husband's mood, disposition, and feeling, and assures the futures of her children."[1]

—Jacques DeLangre

CIVILIZATIONS HAVE HISTORICALLY understood that the women in a society are responsible for much of the final food preparation. The men, as providers, do the preliminary work in harvesting, hunting, or purchasing the food. In the Bible, men would grow the crops and raise the herds, and women would typically serve the food. This is in keeping with the God-ordained roles of men being the leaders, and women the helpers—of men going out into the field, and women keeping the home. Actually, the word "lady" is derived from Old English words that mean "loaf-kneader." Ladies have typically been in charge of the making and distributing of bread to their households. The excellent preparation of food is truly the mark of a lady.

The Bible contains many examples of women serving food. To name a few, Sarah served a meal to the angels that visited Abraham; Rebekah prepared the goat for Jacob to bring to Isaac; the Shunamite woman prepared food for Elisha; Jael served buttermilk to Sisera; Abigail brought a large repast to King David and his men; the woman of Proverbs 31 brought her food from afar and gave it to all her household; Mary and Martha served Jesus in their home; and the apostles were entertained in the homes of godly men and their wives.

Food and meals are much spoken of in the Bible, and in nearly all of the sixty-six books. We are told of the harvests God provided for His people, of meals prepared by women, of spoil taken by the men in warfare, and of feasts enjoyed at meetings, at the forming of covenants, at weddings, and at times of national deliverance. Feasts memorialized special occasions and honored special people. The Church Age commenced with a meal—The Lord's Supper—and it will consummate with a meal—the wedding supper of the Lamb.

Women should be careful stewards of the food that their husbands supply to the family and should honor the desires of their husbands regarding the diet that will be observed. However, health should be an area of concern and deliberate thought for men, even if they entrust the majority of practical application to their wives. So, while there are men who are partial to cooking, and there are many special circumstances, I think it may be said that women are generally in charge of their family's meals.

In her whole foods cookbook, Diane Campbell tells how she replaced her family's diet with whole foods in an effort to restore her husband's health. Successful in this, she then shared her advice and many recipes with others in *Step-by-Step to Natural Food*. Her point that the father must be the leader in the dietary direction of the family is well taken.

> Changing the eating habits of your family will not be an easy job. It takes a lot of work and effort. Each member of the family must do his share. It must be a joint adventure. The father seems to be the key in getting this plan to work. When daddy says that he will try certain foods, then the children will try too. Children copy their parents. If they see you eating natural food and enjoying it, they will want to eat the same thing. What a boost when daddy says, "Honey, this whole wheat cherry cobbler is delicious." What a struggle when a father comes home with a half-gallon of sugary, chemical laden, benzyl acetate [artificial strawberry flavor] ice cream, and tells you, "I just had to have some strawberry ice cream."[2]

As we look more into the health benefits of making meals from scratch, I think it will be obvious why God commands women to manage their homes "lest the word of God be blasphemed." The wife or mother's primary focus is the care of her home and family. Necessary things—family health, beautiful aesthetics, and nurturing of children—are all compromised when the woman's heart is not in her home caring for its environment and inhabitants. While there are many possible activities that are done outside the home, there are many possible repercussions when homes are not first made into havens of nourishment. It does not have to take a lot of time to cook three healthful meals per day, but it does take some attention and foresight. Homemade meals are always best! In light of an unmarried woman's possible future responsibilities, learning how to provide healthful meals for a family and keep a non-toxic home should be a notable element of her education.

Does cooking and eating serve God? The following author, Albert Wolters, shows that every action of the Christian should testify of the gospel's power. Indeed, everyday activities are where we spend most of our time.

By far the largest part of our existence is involved in the stuff of everyday life. We sleep, we work, we eat, we rest, we tell stories, we sing songs, we play games, we get married, we raise our children, we tend the sick, we visit our relatives, we bury and mourn the dead...It is precisely in these ordinary activities that the Christian community is called to witness the gospel. The very shape of our lives needs to be a legible letter speaking of Christ and his rule. When we do explain the gospel, such a verbal presentation should be embedded in the warp and woof of our daily Christian lives which in their integrity testify to God's saving power.[3]

The homemaker can take time to give utmost attention to the nutrition of her family; indeed, that task is integral to this vocational description. Time is required to grow or search out wholesome food at economical prices, to manage the resources and freshness of the pantry's stock, to plan ahead for meal preparation, and to satisfy a growing family. A large responsibility, the making of healthful meals is a weighty matter worthy of the best planning. A woman has the unique ability to direct her family's tastes so that they all come to enjoy wholesome food.

Children seem to have a propensity to crave unhealthy food until they are trained to think about health, especially if their friends are eating something that their parents do not allow. However, children can be perfectly satisfied with the wholesome food that their parents eat, once required to eat it. Too often children avoid vegetables at mealtimes and then ask for—and are given—sugary or refined snacks a couple hours later. Unhealthy food should not be in the house to begin with, but the parents are the true managers of their children's diets and ought to take control. For the sake of the child's further health and the health of the children's children someday, parents should neither give in to constant begging nor think lightly of indulging their children with rich treats. Indulging the child is not loving the child; children must exercise self-discipline in eating just as in other obedience. The best way to guard a child's diet is to provide only permissible things to eat and to teach him to desire those things; otherwise, the sweetest foods will be the most attractive, making it harder for him to desire wholesome foods. If they consider a child's lifelong health before momentary happiness, parents may more easily make the right decisions and require their child to do the same.

From a nineteenth-century English clergyman, John Angell James, comes the following, and very particular, instruction. He emphasizes that parents are ultimately responsible for the children's diet—regardless of the children's appetites or of doting relatives:

Having made these preliminary remarks, I go on to enumerate and illustrate the various branches of parental duty...A due regard to the health of children should be maintained. Physical education is of no small importance...Fond and foolish mothers should be warned against pampering their appetites with sweets, corrupting their blood with grossness, or impairing the tone of their stomachs with fermented liquors. Infanticide is practiced even in this Christian land, by many who never dream that they are child murderers: they do not kill their babes by strangling or poisoning them; no, but by pampering or stuffing them to death. And where they go not to this extreme, they breed up a circle of gluttons, or drunkards. Nothing can be more disgusting than to see children invited to eat all the delicacies of the dinner, and to drink after it the health of the company, with what their young palates ought to be strangers to.

And lamentably injudicious it is to make the gratification of the appetite a reward for good conduct, and to have them ushered into the parlour, before they retire to rest, to receive the luscious sweet, which is the bribe for their going to bed. The mischief goes beyond the corruption of their health, for it brings them up to be governed by appetite, rather than by reason; which is, in fact, the secret cause of all the intemperance and profligacy of the world. Settle your plans on this subject, and suffer neither a favourite servant, nor a kind aunt, nor a doting grandpapa, to come between you and the welfare of your children.[4]

If a family, especially the young children, eats nutritiously, the family will spend less time being sick and the whole family economy can operate more efficiently. Immune systems will be fortified instead of being constantly attacked by unhealthy food, and viruses will descend upon the household with much less frequency. If the children are sick less often, the father is less likely to catch a virus and miss days of work. The health of one person affects not only that individual but also the entire family.

Homemade food is a blessing in numerous ways. If one or more family members spend time away from home working, the mother or wife has the opportunity to prepare nourishing food for their lunches or other meals. Eating in restaurants is expensive and usually not as healthful as the food that can be prepared at home.

The way that food is eaten shapes the culture. To have a fine and civilized culture, the family meal must be given attention. Some places in the world still give more attention to the art of mealtimes than most Americans tend to do. In his book *In Defense of Food*, Michael Pollan compares the unhurried dining culture of the Europeans to the body-fueling eating habits of Americans. The author, a stalwart defender of real food and the art of cuisine, here defends the institution of the family meal.

That one should feel the need to mount a defense of 'the meal' is sad, but then I never would have thought 'food' needed defending, either...It is at the dinner table that we socialize and civilize our children, teaching them manners and the art of conversation. At the dinner table parents can determine portion sizes, model eating and drinking behavior, and enforce social norms about greed and gluttony and waste. Shared meals are about much more than fueling bodies; they are uniquely human institutions where our species developed....this thing we call culture.[5]

Meals eaten together as a family are a place where children are discipled in Christian aesthetics; where the husband can preside as head of the table and relax after a day of work; where the mother can nourish her family with good things; where the whole family can converse; and where the Lord's bountiful gifts can be shared with guests. Beautiful presentation coupled with a loving, personal touch is a combination that can be found at few restaurants. Wholesome meals eaten in the company of family and friends are far different from convenient foods eaten in the car by oneself, though the latter may be necessary on occasion.

William Dufty, author of *Sugar Blues*, makes the following observation, calling the family meal a ceremony:

> In earlier times, the kitchen and the dining area were sacred places in the home. The mother kept the family together by the food she cooked. No other earthly ceremony surpassed it in importance. It is no wonder most American families are fragmented today. In the twentieth century, family could be characterized as a group having the same address and telephone number.[6]

Beautiful meals bless the heart when served in love, but meals must be equally good in quality as in love if they are to nourish the body. A beef steak from a cow fattened in feedlots and kept alive with drugs might serve as a tempting foundation for a spectacular meal, but it can spell disaster in the body. The Proverb about a "jewel of gold in a swine's snout" reminds us of the incongruity of certain things. The integrity of the ingredients must match the purpose of the entire presentation: to fill and nourish the people seated at the table. Making poor choices with good intentions is not good enough; we must become informed about the nutrition quality of the food we serve so that we know it will fit our intentions of nourishment.

While meals are wonderful family events, and while, women typically prepare food, men or women who live alone should still eat healthfully. Cooking simply with wholesome ingredients does not take a lot of time, and restaurants and delicatessens with wholesome food are available for those with little time to eat at home.

The next comparison was quoted in *Nourishing Traditions*. It shows a perceptive observation of changes over a century's span:

> In the 1880's the great majority of Americans ate at home; three family meals a day, homemade, from whole foods. In the 1980's the great majority of Americans do not eat three family meals a day, meals are not normally homemade, and the whole foods are not chosen to any great extent.[7]

Another example of the differences in diets across a hundred-year span is from a White House Cookbook that my dad once brought home for me after a trip to our national capitol. A revision of an 1894 publication, the cookbook was issued as a Centennial edition in 1996, and for modern tastes. The preface explains that "today's diets have changed" and explains the low-fat changes that have updated the nineteenth-century recipes. I agree that today's diets have changed, but they have not changed for the better. Old-fashioned food has been replaced with newfangled food, and bad things have begun to happen—obesity and rampant disease. Instead of going back to the old ways, food industries alter the new ways even more.

Butter from confinement-raised dairy cows is not nearly as healthy as that from pasture-grazed cattle, but the mainstream food industry has not considered the change in raising cattle. Seeing a change in people's weight, industry giants decided to change things even more—with butter substitutes! This White House cookbook uses altered or artificial substitutes for butter, for eggs, and for sugar, and low-fat substitutes for whole-fat dairy products. An old recipe for chocolate macaroons uses melted dark chocolate, eggs, sugar, and butter; the revised version uses cake mix, chocolate frosting, egg substitutes, and partially-hydrogenated canola oil. The 1894 recipe for popcorn balls calls for popcorn kernels, molasses, brown sugar, and vinegar; the 1996 recipe calls for popcorn kernels, marshmallows, and margarine. (I still use the cookbook; I just use the original, old-fashioned ingredients instead!)

Another recipe that I saw in a magazine was titled as "a deceptively good-for-you dessert." Reading the ingredients, I thought—"*deceptive* is right." The raspberry sherbet, the fat-free milk, the sugar-free instant pudding, and the non-dairy whipped topping called for are all loaded with artificial and refined ingredients: sweeteners, colors, flavors, corn syrup, and hydrogenated oil. "Deceptive" was right—all of the products contained artificial ingredients, and none of them good for you. There is *nothing* natural in this recipe; the milk is the closest to something natural, but it is fat-free, not to mention homogenized and pasteurized. Whatever happened to real cream and real raspberries, reminiscent of English teatime? Artificial ingredients might deceive the purchaser, but they will not deceive the human body. The body will react, since it instinctively knows the difference, even if our minds do not know or react.

In conventional nutrition, black has become white and white, black. A recent diet craze has been to manufacture low-fat versions of any possible food, yet people carry more extra weight than ever before. Rather than looking at the healthy nature of another century's diets (when people thrived on real butter, clean red meat, and cold-pressed oils), or rather than looking at the unhealthy nature of today's manufactured oils, people gravitate toward processed fats and artificial sweeteners as their solution to unwanted pounds. Not only do major industries and associations push artificial ingredients as the path toward health, but many magazines and cookbooks marketed to the traditional home cook also push the same ingredients as supposedly nourishing for the family. The image portrayed in many illustrations is that of cooking good meals at home just like families have always done; yet the ingredients called for will have exactly the opposite effect. (I should note—there are many good magazines and cookbooks geared toward natural from-scratch cooking, whether simple or gourmet, that are quite useful and inspiring for home cooks. These are worth searching out.)

Most people, including Christians, have not studied their history to see how far we have left the traditions and practices of our great-grandparents. The more removed we get from the source of food, and from the kitchen and the dining table, the less we will notice the unfortunate changes that are happening.

The kitchen used to be the center of the home—the place of fellowship and nourishment. While the kitchen is often still called the center of the home, it often is not. The microwave, refrigerator, and trashcan, in many American homes, have replaced the cook stove, the pantry, and the dining table. As Sally Fallon Morell has said in *Nourishing Traditions*, the whole family "needs to get back into the kitchen" where food is "prepared with wisdom and love." Truly, both ideas are fundamental to family meals: knowing what we are preparing and eating—and serving it with care for the health and well-being of a spouse and children.

> Blessed is every one that feareth the LORD; that walketh in his ways. For thou shalt eat the labour of thine hands: happy shalt thou be, and it shall be well with thee. Thy wife shall be as a fruitful vine by the sides of thine house: thy children like olive plants round about thy table. Behold, that thus shall the man be blessed that feareth the LORD.
>
> —Psalm 128:1–4

I encourage you to have *Nourishing Traditions* in your kitchen and to study the work of Dr. Weston Price, Dr. Mary Enig, and Sally Fallon Morell. This tome is a foundational resource in what is known as traditional and nutritional eating. In their volume, they boldly call modern food conventions what they are and call us back to walk in life-giving old paths—though not from a distinctly Christian perspective. They reveal incredible information about isolated communities where men and women regularly lived to over one hundred years old, and where childbirth was uncomplicated. Is not the following piece from the preface to *Nourishing Traditions*, from which writing I have learned much, a noble purpose? Fads are measured up against traditions, and compromise is measured up against history.

The premise of this book is that modern food choices and preparation techniques constitute a radical change from the way man has nourished himself for thousands of years and, from the perspective of history, represent a fad that not only has severely compromised his health and vitality but may well destroy him...

Studies too numerous to count have confirmed Dr. Price's observations that the so-called civilized diet, particularly the Western diet of refined carbohydrates and devitalized fats and oils, spoils our God-given genetic inheritance of physical perfection and vibrant health...Technology can be a kind father but only in partnership with his mothering, feminine partner—the nourishing traditions of our ancestors.[8]

"Traditional peoples" or "traditional diets" means eating what people groups could hunt, gather, or raise; this was done for thousands of years up until, or despite of, the advent of modern technology in Western Civilization and Western export of food and dietary practices to third world countries. Barring famines and war, God has provided food wherever people groups have settled—or they settled where food was—and that food has shaped cultures and nourished families for millennia. There were few places in need of the West's processed food until the present time in history; and why now? God's Word repeatedly promises that He will give food to all His creation, and He has always done so.

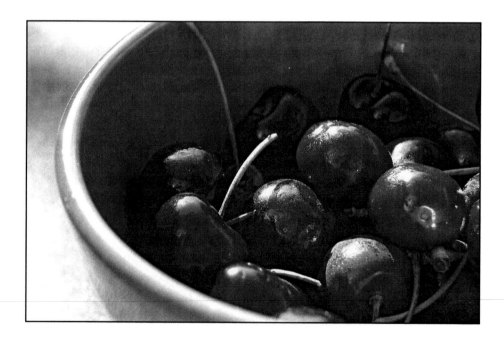

Chapter Twelve

Some European Trends

"God be merciful unto us, and bless us; and cause his face to shine upon us; Selah.
That thy way may be known upon earth, thy saving health among all nations. Then
shall the earth yield her increase; and God, even our own God, shall bless us. God
shall bless us; and all the ends of the earth shall fear him."

—Psalm 67:1–2, 6–7

T HE EUROPEAN CONTINENT, including the United Kingdom, is the source of much of our American heritage—ancestrally, religiously, politically, and culturally. We can still learn from Europe, a region which in many ways is still steeped in her past, being surrounded by it. America's Western expansion moved beyond her first places of settlement, often moving beyond it ideologically as pioneers sought fresh, uncharted territory. Europe, however, has built around and among her monuments to the past and, in some ways, is still influenced by it. In health and in nutrition, at least, Europe has generally held onto more-natural practices and has rejected the modern conventions pushed forward in the United States.

Because they are more steeped in history than Americans are, Europeans seem wary of the newest innovations in food manufacturing. European countries have banned genetically-modified foods and resist using hormones in dairy and meat products. Americans have developed preservative- and oil-laden processed cheese that is ready-sliced and melts easily, but Europeans make wheels of hard cheeses that cure for months, even years, to gain the best flavor. In their cuisine, Europeans have a good sense of what is enduring and are willing to use time-honored methods rather than plunging after the latest ideas. We should use godly principles to discern—and eat—the best things that our culture makes possible.

European cuisine is widely thought superior to American cuisine, and this could be why: it preserves the natural tastes of food and uses long methods of preparation, including aging. Europeans are patient and willing to take time, in both cooking and eating, whereas Americans are always in a hurry. Italians are willing to wait thirty years to open a flask of aged balsamic vinegar, yet many Americans do not even want to take the time to cook with it. Europeans seem to eat similar foods as Americans but in more wholesome versions, and therefore contract much less heart disease. They eat a lot of fat, but in the heart-healthy forms of monounsaturated olive oil, raw milk, antibiotic-free cheese, and good, clean, natural butter. Europeans spend a larger percentage of their income (fourteen to seventeen percent) on food than do Americans (nine to ten percent)—another indicator of the importance Europeans place on quality and sustenance.[1]

Dr. Ben Lerner comments on the noteworthy paradox in which Europeans love feasting on "rich and fattening food" as much as or more than Americans do, yet Americans are the ones with much higher rates of obesity and heart disease. The difference must be in the quality of food eaten, not in the categories of food eaten or the amount of food eaten, he suggests:

> The excessive obesity and the extremely high rate of nutritionally related diseases in Western society is related less to how much food Americans eat than to what is done to those foods. Health problems caused by food in the United States are mostly due to the fact that a high percentage of the American diet is made up of highly refined convenient and fast foods. These foods are prepared with an abundance of chemicals, additives, and preservatives, many of which are not even allowed in other parts of the world [i.e. Europe].[2]

Europeans definitely know how to make food—from cheese to chocolate. Anyone who has tasted croissants or éclairs from a French patisserie—pastry shop—knows they are incomparable. Croissants (my favorite occasional food, admittedly) are made with fine flour, but in Europe the wheat is not genetically modified and the butter is produced without hormones. With a bakery in every village or on every city street, pastries never need to be preserved for shipment across the country.

Though the fine foods of European restaurants are healthier than their American counterparts, and though many people love the charm of Old World cities, with good reason, the mountains cannot be rivaled for the health that they nurture. Dr. Weston Price studied, among many other settlements worldwide, the diets of the families living in Switzerland's mountain villages. The cattle were grazed on pure, verdant grass, and their raw milk was made into cheeses to last through the winter. Bread was made from whole grains. The mountain people were some of the healthiest that Dr. Price found in his world travels; they were of good stature with strong bones and teeth and little disease.[3]

An example of the mountain lifestyle is found in the classic literature story *Heidi* by Johanna Spyri. Klara, an invalid living in the city, became well when she visited and experienced the crisp mountain air and ate the dark rustic bread, fresh goat's milk, and wholesome raw-milk cheese from the Grandfather's table. We know Klara had a richer, less healthful diet in Frankfurt since Heidi had brought back soft white rolls for Peter's grandmother on the mountain. It is no wonder Heidi ached to return to the mountain. Based on her diet in both places, Heidi probably felt much better in the alpine hut. There she enjoyed strengthening food and the invigorating exercise of frolicking with Peter and the goatherd.

While European bakery goods are appealing to the eye and, with their time-intensive preparation and real ingredients, are a mainstay of the European diet, other parts of European cuisine are the points we should especially emulate. Europeans do not feel the need to make food unnatural. For instance, they neither irradiate nor modify food, nor inject cattle with drugs. They will not give hormones and antibiotics to chickens or cattle. Since Americans do inject drugs into our animals, as Dr. Jordan Rubin states, "the European Common Market refuses to import livestock from American farms."[4]

Following is an example from the World War II era showing the difference between European and American ideas of what constitutes good bread. The British loaves were federally required to be mostly whole grain, while American bakers catered to what they thought people wanted (refined bread) and then added back in enough vitamins to meet federal requirements. Also, the following quote gives insight into an interesting equalizing factor of industrialization—the poor (assumedly in cities)now have access to better food, but that same selection of food is worse than what the rich were accustomed to eating. From James Trager's *The Food Chronology*:

> Britain's rich do not eat as well as they did before the war, but the poorer third of the population enjoys better nutrition than it has in decades. British bakers are required to make the 'national loaf,' made up about 85 percent of whole wheat flour, partly as a means of providing the nutrients found in enriched U.S. white bread; U.S. authorities find it more reasonable to restore certain food factors to the refined bread and cereal products that people want.[5]

Earlier, again, in the twentieth century, Dr. Weston Price also studied Scottish and Irish farmers and fisherman in the northern parts of those countries. They were, like the Swiss mountain people, specimens of robust health. Whenever they moved to cities, however, or were otherwise influenced by a more refined diet, their health began to decline and their teeth began to decay.

Before the Industrial Revolution, the staple food of the Scottish nation was oats. Known today as a super-food, oats was the dietary basis undergirding the nation that has taken its place in history for confidence and stalwartness. In folklore, as well as in the testimony of science, oats are credited with lending beauty, perceptiveness, strength, and endurance to the men and women who consume them, even to soldiers on the battlefield. Based on what we know of the health benefits of oats and what we know of the historical achievements of Scotland—if ever a food made a nation, this is a prime example. A food so commonly used, such as oats were in Scotland, would be typically used in combination with a complementary protein food such as fish.

Wholesome foods eaten with complementary proteins or starches are vastly unlike the recent American emphasis on single foods, for example, soy. Whereas soy contributes to Asian health (where fermented soy products are eaten along with seafood, vegetables, and sea vegetables) Americans usually eat genetically-modified soy in the worst possible combinations: with refined flours and trans-fats in processed foods. A "staple" food used in this way will be detrimental, causing more ruin than good in the body since the food is not well balanced for optimal benefit. God's foods are usually eaten in combination with one another. Other recent emphases in health foods have been oat bran and wheat germ. While these products and others may be good supplements, they do not take the place of consuming quantities of whole foods such as the Scottish people did with their oats.

In his research, Dr. Price noted the drastic change in health resulting from diets of industrialized people groups. Though the more northerly British people had once been prime specimens of health, the English have not been known for their good health ever since the sugar industry bloomed in the eighteenth century. The royalty, who had often been most healthful (and therefore often renowned for their beauty) due to obtaining the best foods available, were now able to afford the latest in imported foods: cane sugar.

Major villains in the history of the British Empire and Western Civilization were the slave trade and sugar trade, both of which were based on greed and proved to be destructive. The British love of sugar tracks the general trend toward unhealthfulness common to industrialized nations; however, Britain, along with the rest of Europe, has been wary of many American conventions, even denying their use or importation.

As William Dufty documents in *Sugar Blues*, drastic and noticeable affects appeared *"after sugar made the transition from apothecary's prescription to candy maker's confection.... after sugar consumption in Britain had zoomed in two hundred years from a pinch or two in a barrel of beer here and there to more than two million pounds per year. By that time, physicians in London had begun to observe and record terminal physical signs and symptoms of the sugar blues.*"[6]

While Europe certainly has not held on to her roots in every sphere, becoming more socialist and post-Christian all the time, she has researched trends which America seems to ignore. Scientific findings, such as direct sunlight for pregnant mothers strengthens the bones of babies in the womb, or that cell phones are seriously harmful for children to use, tend to come from British, Scandinavian, and Australian universities. Europeans are more committed with their euros than Americans are with their dollars in supporting the organic industry. America needs to respect her past, regarding the standards even of modern Europe—instead of deeming ourselves more revolutionary and advanced than the rest of the world.

Chapter Thirteen

Our Natural Environment

"Though nothing can bring back the hour, Of splendor
in the grass, of glory in the flower..."[1]

—William Wordsworth

"We will not grieve but rather find
New wealth, new health, new paradigms;
The time is ripe and not too late
For splendid herbs and splendid yields
And splendid children born of splendid fields."[2]

—Wordsworth, rewritten anonymously for the present time

THE ENVIRONMENT GOD created is not only the source of all good food but also has innumerable benefits the closer our lives are connected with it. Health is promoted by being in fresh, country air and direct, clear sunshine—more so than any manmade air conditioning, heat, or lighting. Living in a place where we can see, appreciate, and enjoy the natural world helps us to consider our lifestyle's relation to the environment more than does being detached from the environment by living in a large metropolis of manmade conditions. God's creation and our lives are closely intertwined; everything that we use to live comes from the earth. Realizing this association and being surrounded by natural reminders of it will help us to be better stewards of the earth and our bodies. So much of creation helps us to understand life, and we should not be removed from these lessons. Yet, nature is only general revelation to all mankind, and we need God's Word to inform our interaction with it.

Two extremes of lifestyles exist in the world that God has made and man has developed. One pattern is to live very close to nature, secluded from other people, with the intent to be self-sufficient. This lifestyle can inhibit the ability for commercial trade, Christian fellowship, and cultural impact.

Another pattern is to live much removed from nature in the middle of a city and to seldom venture beyond it. This lifestyle can inhibit the ability to enjoy God's creation, to receive health benefits from fresh air, and to know the source of our food (and it's not the store).

The Old Testament Israelites were mainly an agrarian people, yet the New Testament was addressed to churches in cities. The world began with a garden, as we read in the book of Genesis, but it will end with a city, as we read in the book of Revelation. "And the LORD God planted a garden eastward in Eden; and there he put the man whom he had formed" (Gen. 2:8). ... "And he carried me away in the spirit to a great and high mountain, and shewed me that great city, the holy Jerusalem, descending out of heaven from God" (Rev. 21:10).

A biblical case cannot, therefore, be made for either rural or urban living; yet I think it can be said that with today's busy cities, extra care is needed to avoid pollution from transportation and manufacturing, contamination of drinking water, radiation from electronics, and toxicity from chemicals that are used in practically every space and on every surface. A place where you have more determination over your environment, or a place where God's environment is left as it is, can be more advantageous in the care of our health.

Keeping in mind the extremes of rarely experiencing communities, or of rarely experiencing nature, where we live does not much matter as long as we follow God's commandments. If we take good care of our bodies and invest in the health of future generations, as well as taking time for serving other people in our families, churches, and communities, we can live anywhere. Most importantly, we should have a biblical perspective well thought out and well lived out, regarding where we place our residence and what we do with ourselves there.

City life is not inferior; community living is very well developed there, as are possibilities for the many things we are divinely commanded to do culturally and socially, religiously and politically. Other places may be accessed by transportation, but if a family lives in the country without going to the city, or lives in the city without going to the country, neither is prudent. Both agrarian and community lifestyles are shown favor in God's Word. The point remains that we need to understand God's world—wherever we live—and connect to it in a manner that our health and welfare are increased. Our lives are dependent upon nature whether we live in the midst of the natural world or in the city, and we do well to remain aware of this truth since it becomes less obvious the more we are surrounded by industrialism.

Culture and society are good and God-ordained things, but they are always in essence "religion externalized." The author of *Creation Regained* emphasizes that creation was designed to be developed. As an earlier quotation from the same book noted, all of God's world has fallen and is characterized by sin, and all must eventually be transformed by Christ's redemption.

> One should not think that the scriptural emphasis on restoration implies that Christians should advocate a return to the Garden of Eden, however. We have already noted that creation develops through culture and society and that this development is good and healthy. Part of God's plan for the earth is that it be filled and subdued by humankind, that its latent possibilities be unlocked and actualized in human history and civilization. A good deal of that has already taken place, though it is distorted by humanity's sinfulness.[3]

People can live in a way consumed with popular culture while they live out in the country; or they can make their city plot into a verdant garden. Location is not virtuous of itself. While living closer to nature is not more spiritual, that kind of lifestyle does allow us to better benefit from the beauty of nature. In town or country life, large quantities of food can be raised and grown economically. Men and women used to be knowledgeable about healing herbs, homemade remedies, and such, but the past generations have left this behind as they have flocked to population centers. The more detached we are from nature, the more we rely on popular culture's interpretation of nature.

A recent article from the United Kingdom gave statistics on the minimal time that school children spent outdoors. The parents and teachers were rightly concerned that these would be the children stewarding the environment in the next generation, and the parents were lamenting the children's ill-preparedness.

I remember hearing my mom speak of growing up in Los Angeles. The mountain range was quite close to their home, but she often could not see it due to smog. Some city dwellers would go years without seeing any livestock. My dad grew up in the city, too, near San Francisco, but made every effort during high school and college to be out in the country. He would go backpacking, camping, and hiking in city, state, and national parks every chance he could. He started a conservation club on his college campus, as well as becoming involved in numerous outdoor-minded organizations. Once he graduated, he rented a house surrounded by almond orchards because he loved the fragrance and the atmosphere. After my parents married, they moved to Montana where they loved the accessibility of the mountains and the wide open spaces.

Other than two brief times, our family has always lived on pieces of property, sometimes on large acreages and always out of town. We have raised cattle, have hunted elk, deer, and antelope, and have grown our own vegetable garden and berry patch to supply us with a year's worth of food. We had a tree farm as a business for a number of years that gave us much experience in physical labor and a great education in botany. My brother and I never needed a play-set in the backyard, for we had twenty acres of grassy hillsides, rocky outcroppings, and juniper trees to explore. We practically spent whole summers outdoors with one activity or another.

One of the main pleasures of the outdoors is the gift of sunshine. I love sunshine! I am writing this book in the winter, waiting for summer to come. While we get exercise during the winter and seldom get sick during that time, we *never* get sick in the summer. By spending time in the sunshine and getting exercise, everything in our bodies seems to feel better and work better. Sunshine sanitizes and exercise energizes!

Sunshine, fresh air, and exercise are so very healthful and cannot be re-created by indoor gyms or by pictures of the outdoors. Where people used to do old-fashioned hard work outdoors, people now tend to hide from the sun and exercise indoors, if at all. What has happened?

The sun brightens our spirits. In fact, vitamin D is called the "sunshine vitamin" and a deficiency of it contributes to melancholy and lethargy. Just being out in the sun always makes me happy, and bright summer days render low spirits improbable. Most people that get cancer have had vitamin D deficiencies; proper levels of vitamin D slash cancer risk by seventy-five percent. Sunshine is the most beneficial source of vitamin D; there are few other natural sources of this vitamin.

Dr. Joseph Mercola believes that sun exposure is vital for optimum wellbeing, but that many people are "dangerously deficient" in, specifically, the vitamin D which comes so profusely and freely from the sun's rays. He relates that in the past forty years, the medical community has made an extreme reaction to the matter of UV rays and most people have made an extreme reaction to the sun—evading it altogether.[4]

Sunshine creates energy in plants and strength in humans. Animals fed on healthy plants are the most nutritious for people to eat; grass-fed and wild animals usually live in the sunshine. Sunshine is important for pregnant women in order for their babies to have strong bones. (Summer babies are, on average, taller and stronger than winter-born babies.) People who have been out in the sunshine during the day will sleep better at night.

Though the benefits of sunshine are countless, prolonged exposure can burn our skin. How can we protect ourselves from getting too much sun at one time? From living in a temperate mountain climate and having always tanned easily, I am not very knowledge-able on how to survive with fair skin in a subtropical climate. It is true, however, that people never used to use sunscreen. Gradual exposure to more sun, as spring arrives, is the greatest protection. As the skin tans, a barrier to the sun's harmful rays is formed. Many sunscreens are harmful and are even said to cause skin cancer. If you have to use sunscreen, purchase an organic type without chemical UV-absorbers or preservatives and containing good oils that will nourish and protect the skin—and use it sparingly.

Our diets actually contribute to sunburn. New-fangled hydrogenated oils used in most prepared foods do not protect our skin like natural oils do; they compromise the body's natural ability. God wisely provided olives as native plants in the warm Mediterranean climate, and coconuts as native plants in sunny tropical climates. The oils from both of these plants nourish the skin. Coconut oil, especially, gives protection against the sun. Also, many garden vegetables eaten in season during midsummer, such as tomatoes, protect the skin against damage. We should eat the good, natural things God created and not be fearful of the sun which God has provided for the earth's light, warmth, and sustenance. "Without whole food," says one doctor, "sunshine's ultraviolet light has a greater chance of damaging the skin."[5]

Sugar in our bloodstreams also affects our reception of sunshine, as reported by William Dufty. Interestingly, the very time many people tend to eat sugary beverages is while laboring under the hot sun, with the view that such drinks will replenish energy.

> After you've kicked sugar for a year or so, you begin to notice big changes in the way your skin takes to the sun. Sitting in the hot sun covered with chemical sauce to get a beautiful tan is looking for trouble—especially for women. After you've kicked sugar you will discover that *sunbathing without any protective lotion is* usually possible with little or no risk of burning or peeling.[6]

The benefits of coconuts and coconut oil for skin protection are worthy of further mention. Rubbing coconut oil directly into the skin can be a natural tanning agent and is something I have often done before a long period of time outdoors. Polynesians have used this proven technique for centuries, but modern industries try to convince people that the reverse is true: that both coconut oil and sunshine are harmful. Modern wisdom has produced dire consequences in heart disease and skin cancer; should we not rather consider ancient wisdom? Dr. Bruce Fife presents the fascinating combination of facts that Polynesian islanders wear a small amount of clothing, are exposed to the sweltering sun, and have beautiful blemish-free and cancer-free skin. He views the properties of coconut oil to be a main reason for this, saying:

> The difference between coconut oil and other creams and lotions is that the latter are made to bring immediate, temporary relief. Coconut oil, on the other hand, not only brings quick relief but also aids in the healing and repairing process.[7]

In *The Coconut Oil Miracle*, the above author explains exactly why and how the above relief and healing happens, and gives many accounts of the oil's wonders for people suffering from assorted skin conditions. I can testify to the worth of coconut oil, as well, in a very arid climate—as can many people who have used the coconut oil lotion that I have made and sold at farmers' markets. Where expensive laboratory-formulated skin products fall short, simple coconut oil gives unparalleled performance, yet another testament to God's wisdom surpassing that of man.

Being outdoors or being reminded of the outdoors are both calming and relaxing, which confirms the perception that green is the most comfortable color to look at and that blue is a peaceful, harmonizing color. Our lives are sustained by plants that grow outdoors under the sky, and by animals that eat growing things, so it follows that we should be interested in nature and soothed by it.

God made the world so that joy and profit can come from several places at once. You can exercise in the city or indoors, but working outside in the unpolluted sunshine and raising natural foods while gazing at mountains or vistas allows multi-tasking and multiplies immeasurable benefits upon us.

A Californian transplanted to a Virginia farm commented about his experience growing to love a simpler lifestyle and respecting God's creation more than man's developments: "We are learning to reject Modernism's worship of science and technology; and we are realizing that nature is a gift of amazing beauty, resilience, and wealth."[8]

While mankind can invent and is designed to invent many items of wonder and cultural development, nothing surpasses the beauty of God's earth. We would do well to spend time in nature, respect God's wisdom seen in it, and reference it in all our technological advancements.

Chapter Fourteen

Surrounded by Pollution

"In an underdeveloped country, don't drink the water; in
a developed country, don't breathe the air."[1]

—Jonathan Raban

IN ADDITION TO the environment surrounding our home, another important aspect of a healthy lifestyle is the environment *inside* our home. The air outside might be clean, but the air inside makes a big difference as well. Have you heard the term "non-toxic home"?[2] Houses, as well as soil or food, can be full of toxins. It is in our best interest to eliminate these toxins. The most obvious items to pay attention to and replace are any non-food consumable products that are brought into our homes. While it is incredibly hard and expensive to build or remodel a house with environmentally-friendly products, this can be done and is probably very wise. As most of us are not in a financial position to build with "green" products, I will concentrate on the steps that are more feasible.

While practically everything manufactured is produced with dyes and chemicals, the things that generally end up causing allergies and that are the most dangerous to our health are those products that contain either fragrances or consumable liquid. Breathing in and absorbing chemicals lessens immunity and renders people more susceptible to viruses and diseases. Dr. Don Colbert has made the cautionary and rather comprehensive statement that "dangerous chemicals are everywhere."[3]

Many people are developing multiple-chemical-sensitivity and have to stay away from anything that can cause an allergic reaction. With all of the fragrances used in manufacturing, it would be no surprise if this malady becomes a lot more common.

Whatever you become desensitized to will go unnoticed, but as soon as you are removed from it and come back, it can become very noticeable. After trying to stay away from chemical fragrances and cleaners, I notice that the smell starts to irritate me when I am around fragrances again. While some people are more sensitive than others, I think we should not excuse the potential for harm; chemicals are foreign to our bodies and we should stay away from them. As one example, some research indicates that the use of chemical fragrances is even linked to deficient thyroid production—and deficient thyroid production is linked to countless health problems.

The following advice is from the vigilant work of Debra Lynn Dadd, who has long researched the detrimental effects of toxic chemicals. Exact evidence is only slowly becoming known and published, but more broadly, the evidence supports the fact that "cancer is caused by exposure to toxic chemicals." Sadly, both chemicals and cancer are only becoming more prevalent. Pay attention to her point that chemicals poison all of us whether or not we notice it. I appreciate the reference to how long Ms. Dadd has been conducting her research, as well as her caution regarding *long-term* chemical effects. I am so thankful for the people who have diligently conducted research when it was not widely accepted (it still isn't) and when the evidence was more tenuous.

> Remember, the long term health effects of many chemicals are unknown. We do not know the possible synergistic reactions that occur when chemicals are combined in food, water, or air, or when the chemicals are in your body interacting with other chemicals... While there are certainly some people who are more sensitive to household pollutants than others, it is important to remember that these substances are poisoning all of us, whether or not we feel the effects immediately. Some toxins poison instantly; others show their devastating effects only after years of everyday exposure.

> At the time [that she first sounded the alarm] my claims were viewed with some trepidation by the medical community, but now, almost twenty years later, science is catching up with anecdotal evidence... Since my books were first published, the neurotoxic effects of common household chemicals have become widely known. Neurotoxins are so called because they are toxic to your nervous system. The core of your nervous system is your brain, which not only affects thinking and feeling but regulates every system in your body...And what are these neurotoxic substances? Many of the same petrochemicals that cause [multiple chemical sensitivity] and cancer.[4]

In response, I ask, will we wait until the people who have much at stake *against* the truth about health (financially and politically) actually acknowledge the facts, if they ever do—or will we research and decide for ourselves, and oppose the devastating trends? Ms. Dadd's book, to suggest one resource, recommends and teaches us how to do the latter.

"The effects...have become widely known," she writes. The harmfulness of chemicals is not some obscure bit of documentation that goes against other information. These issues regarding health are widely observed, repeatedly reported on by medical doctors, and all point to one truth: manmade things always contribute to ruin and deterioration, and God-made things always contribute to life and health and joy and peace.

We get bombarded with sensory stimulation too often for our good. Just as a musician would say that having music playing everywhere (banks, stores, and on the radio) does not lend itself to true music appreciation, we are so stimulated by chemical smells that we are not sensitive to genuine smells. For instance, cleaning products are artificially scented; why not open the windows to the blossoming trees outside and get a gentle draft of the real thing? Aren't clean sheets, clean laundry, clean teeth, clean dishes, clean floors, and fresh air enough without having them all scented? People didn't used to clean things with artificial scents. Clean things don't smell bad, so why should they smell like something they are not—fruit, flowers, etc.?

Mankind is, in many ways, more productive than he was one hundred years ago, though progress comes with a cost. The mediums of technology cause major oxidative stress, radiation, and chemical exposure in our bodies. While chemicals are used in the manufacturing of everything from ink to furniture to shampoo, our main area of attention should be what is eaten, what is breathed, and what soaks into the skin—our most direct sources of contact with our environment. Consumable products do one of two things: spread into the air (as in bathroom cleaners) or soak into the skin (as in dish soap or lotion). If products contain chemicals, we either breathe them or absorb them.

Below is a list of substances that are basically household villains, yet they have all been governmentally approved as safe for household use. While pollutants will never destroy the earth (God will see to that), they are still *extremely* dangerous to our health. Christians are supposed to be working for God in restoring the creation, not working against His cause by polluting the earth without thought. Products marketed for convenience usually come with health detriments, but there are natural, simple, and alternative ways to complete the same tasks.

Cleaning, laundry, and dishwashing products: Why would we use a household *cleaning* product plastered with warnings about its danger level and cautions about touching and breathing it? Vinegar, baking soda, borax powder, plain soap, pine oil, lemon juice, peroxide, and water will get just about anything clean and avoid the harm that comes from using chemical cleaners. Many recipe books and cleaning guides exist for maintaining a household with natural products—with many of the products being normal pantry supplies. Conventional laundry powders and dryer sheets are laden with harsh chemicals and harmful chemical fragrances. Conventional dishwashing detergents are poisonous; liquid dish soap has colors, scents, and harmful chemicals that soak into our skin while washing dishes. Organic or natural brands are naturally scented and naturally colored (imagine something left clear!), are made of plant-based materials, and are biodegradable.

While we're talking about laundry, clothing made of natural fibers (cotton, linen, wool, silk, etc.) is healthier to wear, more breathable, less chemical-intensive, and more durable than synthetic fibers. Natural fibers smell better and feel better, besides. Also, wrinkle-free, permanent-press, stain-resistant, and fire-retardant pieces of clothing are treated with chemicals which outgas and which are not good to have against the skin.

Cosmetic, hair, and skincare products: While it used to be believed that skin is impervious, it is now known that the skin soaks in the properties of literally everything on its surface. For this reason, we ought to be very careful about what we put on our skin and in our hair. For example, most deodorants contain aluminum, the absorption of which is believed to lead to Alzheimer's disease. Aerosol hairsprays, antidandruff shampoos, and hair removing lotions are other equally hazardous products. Many liquid hand soaps have harmful chemicals in them, similar to conventional dish soap, yet many people use them to wash their hands and face.

An authority on the subject, Dr. Don Colbert, calls for much prudence in the area of personal products. Many more persuasive details may be found in his book *What You Don't Know May Be Killing You.* Eating right is not enough, since contact with "the most poisonous ingredients in existence" is more toxic than eating the worst foods. The strong words this doctor uses below are appropriate considering the jeopardy that chemicals cause in our bodies.

> The perils of personal products can silently undermine the safety of your home. Without your knowledge, poisons and cancer-causing substances can be absorbed slowly over time through your skin and lungs, and they can accumulate in your body. Some personal and home products are made from some of the most poisonous ingredients in existence. You can eat right, exercise, take supplements, and do everything you know to live healthy, and still be filling your body and the bodies of your loved ones with dangerous poisons. What you don't know about the products you use may be killing you and your family...

> Personal care products and common household chemicals often contain an alphabet soup of chemicals and solvents. We are rubbing chemicals on our faces, applying them

to our skin, spraying them on our hair, using them to wash our hands and clothes and cleaning our homes with them. What is the harm? We are becoming toxic. Over time, the solvents found in personal care products and household products may collect in our central nervous systems, in our tissues and in our organs.[5]

There is a wide range of natural skin and hair products, such as natural cosmetics, deodorants, shampoos, soaps, and more—some of them more natural than others. These products usually contain many fruits and herbs and natural extracts and oils. Choose from companies which list the ingredients they intentionally leave out, such as petrochemicals, parabens, sulfates, and phthalates. Some nutritionists believe that ingredients such as phenols, glycols, and EDTA are also harmful, but these can be found even in products from organic-type companies. Be cautioned that the terms "natural" or "herbal" or "fruity" on conventional-brand products mean basically nothing about the product's health benefits or purity.

Many recipe books exist whereby you can make your own hair rinses, bath salts, body creams, tanning lotions, colognes, baby powders, skin-nourishing soaps, and any other products normally purchased. Most often, these concoctions use typical pantry and refrigerator ingredients, nutrient-rich fruits and vegetables, and health-giving oils—and they rival anything commercially-made.

Feminine napkins and baby diapers: Feminine care products and disposable baby products are bleached with dioxins—one of the most hazardous chemicals known to mankind. Yet, such products are used against tender and susceptible areas of the skin and are known to contribute to cancers of women's reproductive organs. Disposable or non-disposable (i.e. organic cotton) alternatives for all of these products are readily available and strongly recommended.

Miscellaneous scented and medicated products: The air we breathe goes into our blood and then to every cell in our body; it needs to be pure.[6] Candles, aerosol air fresheners, toothpaste, breath fresheners, cough drops, tissues, and toilet paper are prime culprits for chemical fragrances. Any kind of aerosol spray leaves little particles in the air that make their way into our lungs. Candles exude their chemical fragrance whether they are burning or not; the burning of paraffin candles releases petroleum-based carcinogens into the air. (Soy or beeswax candles are cleaner-burning.) While I am used to a clean, artificial-scent-free house, in some houses I have noticed, and am affected by, fragrance in everything from tissues and toilet paper to dryer sheets, potpourri, and candles—and I am probably forgetting some items. Chemicals are found all over houses and grocery stores, and we need to make a determined effort to avoid purchasing or using them.

Without having to get chemical or medication-based cough drops and throat lozenges, you can use a natural herbal type that accomplishes the same task. Much toothpaste has chemical breath fresheners and contains artificial flavors, colors, and even sugar. It is advantageous to buy natural brands that use herbs as disinfectants. Why freshen your breath with a breath strip made with hydroxypropyl methylcellulose, triacetin, flavor, modified corn starch, polysorbate 80, ethyl alcohol, sucralose, and potassium acesulfame—actual ingredients—when you can freshen breath with a lozenge made with organic peppermint oil in a base of molasses and evaporated cane juice?

For years, my family has been using an economical and powdery alternative to toothpaste—a tooth powder made of baking soda and arrowroot powder. When we occasionally travel, we use a non-fluoride toothpaste. The evidence against fluoride is staggering, and here is one opinion from a well-respected medical doctor, Dr. Mercola:

> The risks of fluoride far outweigh any benefit. Fluoride is more toxic than lead and is used as a pesticide for mice, rats, and other small pests...Indeed, fluoride has been linked to cancer and to weakened bones and osteoporosis.[7]

As shown above, the same chemicals used in small amounts for personal care or consumption, such as fluoride in toothpaste, are used in large and caustic amounts for more powerful tasks, such as fluoride in pesticide. In chapter seventeen, poison is discussed as being anything that is known to be dangerous in concentration. In diluted or small quantity, however, there are many poisonous substances allowed in our foods and cosmetic products.

Microwave ovens: So much alarming information is available on microwaves that I need not repeat it all here. Microwaves change the molecular structure of food and consequently change how our bodies assimilate and digest food. Microwaves cause free-radicals in the air, especially directly in front of the appliance. (Sensitive people, such as myself, can feel the waves if standing in front of the microwave or even in the same room.) What are free-radicals? Though they are not the extreme political group they might sound like, they are likewise an unwelcome foe to our well-being. Free-radicals are unstable molecules that result in the destruction of living cells. With weakened immune systems already, the last thing we need in our homes is a free-radical factory! Antioxidants from vitamins and fresh foods are the only things that protect against free-radical damage. Getting sufficient antioxidants is difficult as it is without utilizing an attack mechanism—microwaves. Everything that is cooked or heated in a microwave can be prepared on a gas stovetop or in a small toaster oven. Softening butter is the only thing that I have found is hard to duplicate on the stove, but planning ahead or setting the butter in a pan of lukewarm water are good alternatives. The best way to stop using a microwave is to eliminate it from your home and simply use an alternate method.

Aluminum and non-stick cookware: Not only are aluminum pans poor conductors of heat, and therefore shunned by gourmet chefs, but they leach aluminum into food. Aluminum buildup in the body is known to contribute to Alzheimer's and other diseases. Aluminum, highly toxic, is found in conventional baking powder (buy organic to avoid this), non-dairy creamers, processed cheese, refined table salt, cookware, foil, cans, and antiperspirants.[8]

Non-stick cookware is another villain if there ever was one! The perfluorooctanoic acid (PFOA) used in the coating of non-stick cookware is highly toxic to both humans and animals (and lethal for pet birds) when it outgases. PFOA coating releases poisonous fumes at 450-500 degrees, a temperature which is easily reached on high heat when sautéing and frying. PFOAs have been found in tests of human blood, mother's milk, and newborn babies; this chemical is believed to cause tumors and to alter hormones and bodily organs. The Environmental Protection Agency has PFOA listed as a likely human carcinogen, yet it is still in widespread use in manufacturing. Research it more if you like, but please decide to stop using any pans containing it! Stainless steel, glass, and cast iron are the best materials for cooking and are very versatile on the stove top, oven, or toaster oven. For an alternative solution to regular non-stick pans, numerous environmentally-friendly non-stick pans are available which have ceramic coatings, diamond coatings, or enamel-coated cast iron. Professional gourmet cooks do not use convenient types of cookware and heating devices, but take the time to use the best.

Plastic: The softer the plastic, the more it outgases chemicals which then leach into food and into our bodies. Phthalates are chemicals used to soften plastic and are particularly toxic; they mimic hormones and have become known as "gender-benders." Phthalates are present in plastic food storage containers, shower curtains, and even cell phone screens. Soft plastic will outgas even more of its unhealthy composition when it is heated in the microwave (which you just disposed of) or washed in the dishwasher (for which you are now using organic detergent, right?). Glass is the best medium for food storage as it can go from fridge to oven, does not absorb odors or stains, and looks decisively more elegant. Metal, wood, and ceramic are the best options for dinnerware and utensils. Unlike plastic, these mediums do not stain, outgas, absorb odors, or get cuts and cracks that harbor bacteria. While it is hard to get away from plastic completely, one can begin by making big changes in the kitchen and smaller changes in the rest of the house.

Of course you will not discard items such as a computer keyboard (which I am using as I type), but you can take many other steps such as replacing your PVC-coated vinyl shower liner with a nylon one and choosing more wooden, cloth, and metal toys for your children. With all the recent recalls of oriental-made children's toys, I would definitely gravitate toward more timeless, earthy mediums in playthings. Stains on wood and coatings on metal are often very chemical-based, but at least those do not outgas as much as plastic does.

Cell phones: "Mobile phones boost brain tumor risk by up to 270 percent on side of brain where phone is held,"[9] one sample headline read. If you do a Google search for the dangers of cell phones or read an alternative health magazine, headlines like the above will grab your attention. The dangers of cell phones are widely proven. Basically, cell phones send out electromagnetic radiation, dangerously heating up one side of your head and leading to the development of burning sensations, mental confusion, aggressively-growing brain tumors, headaches, and other disorders. If a cell phone is turned on and clipped to your belt, the radiation is aimed toward your liver and kidneys. When cell phones are used repeatedly and over a long period of time, the health risks are acute. I am more sensitive than some people—but if I use a cell phone for only ten minutes, the side of my head on which it is held heats up very uncomfortably. Other people may not be as sensitive, but radiation is certainly still occurring. On top of these warnings, cell phones are especially damaging to the developing brains and nerves of children. Because of skull thickness, cell phones heat up a large portion of a child's head in a few minutes of use, whereas a smaller percentage of an adult's head is heated up in the same amount of time.

I cringe to hear people say that their cell phone is their primary phone at home and/or for work. At home, a substitute can easily be used; get a landline and corded telephones. At work, avoid using the cell phone when you can; make personal calls from home. When you do use one in occupations that rely upon it, keep in mind that corded headsets connected to the cell phone are thought, by some, to intensify the radiation. One debatable alternative is a wireless earpiece, in the use of which the cell phone should be placed away from the body. (My brother, who uses a wireless earpiece when he has to use a cell phone, usually places his phone in the console of his truck or on the far end of his desk at work. It is important to keep it away from your body as much as possible.) There are other radiation-canceling solutions advertised—cell phone chips, little pods or ferrite beads to clip onto the headset cord, as well as various types of headsets with hollow tubes instead of wires—and only time will tell whether or not they are healthy to use. Seeing the risks already associated with cell phones is distressing. If industrialized nations keep going in the same direction toward the historically-unprecedented use of convenience electronics, problems will only get worse. The ease of cell phones seems to be a circumstance about which it should be said, "this is too good to be true!" Make a choice now to protect your health.

Electric appliances: We are swimming in a dangerous sea—a sea that we cannot see. Some of it can be prevented, as long as we first become aware of the issues at stake. I only have space to introduce the subject of electromagnetic radiation; its dangers and the research of them are prolific—much too extensive to cover here.

> Every day, we're swimming in a sea of electromagnetic radiation (EMR) produced by electrical appliances, power lines, wiring in buildings, and a slew of other technologies that are part of modern life. From the dishwasher and microwave oven in the kitchen and the clock radio next to your bed, to the cellular phone you hold to your ear—sometimes for hours each day—exposure to EMR is growing and becoming a serious health threat.[10]

The human body has a natural energy field and manmade electromagnetic fields disrupt the natural protection that God gave us, altering it and weakening it. Electromagnetic fields enter that natural barrier that surrounds our bodies, compromising our immune systems and leading to the greatest rise in immune system disorders in history. We live in an "electronic soup" of wiring, lights, appliances, and machines. Getting away from electromagnetic radiation prevalent in cities is one reason to live in the country.

Many choices can be made to cut down on exposure to radiation, since it would be almost impossible to get away from it completely. Sleep, which should fill one-third of our day, is a good time to get completely away from radiation. Sleep in complete darkness. If possible, use heating other than electric heat and never use electric blankets. Do not have a computer in your bedroom, or turn it completely off at night, and keep your alarm clock several feet away from your head.

In other areas of the house, cut down on electric appliances used for every little job, and cut down on electric toys for children. Never leave a charging cord plugged into an outlet if the cord is not plugged into the device. This position creates electromagnetic radiation that can be felt in the room if you are sensitive like I am. I would go unplug my brother's charging cords and instantly my ears would stop ringing and buzzing; I finally convinced him not to leave cords plugged in.

For computers, which seem to be a necessary tool of the age, you can take several actions. Flat panel screens are supposed to have less radiation than convex screens. Ionic lights or ionic candles are supposed to generate beneficial negative ions which counteract the harmful positive ions generated by computers and electronic devices. Fresh air from an open window brings in beneficial negative ions as well.

We are bombarded with radiation even when airborne. "[Wireless internet in airplanes] adds a significant additional source of non-iodizing radiation to the flying environment which is already filled with positively charged ions detrimental to our health. They cause staleness and dryness in the air, and more importantly accelerate oxidation in our bodies...Fliers already have enough to contend with and don't need any technology which makes this challenging environment worse.[11]

It is important to be aware of the damage that comes to our bodies from electromagnetic radiation. For instance, one study found a correlation between Alzheimer's disease and people who lived near power lines. We can begin to make wise choices as we are able and research ways to make larger changes toward a healthier lifestyle. If we understand that radiation is constantly attacking our immune systems, it will be wise to consume as many antioxidant-rich foods as possible, primarily vegetable foods. And yet, we should not think that one little area of nutrition will save us. We need to be vigilant and consistent in every area of our lifestyles.

Other pollutants: In *Home Safe Home*, these are some of the toxic things that Ms. Dadd discusses: automobile exhaust, plastics, electromagnetic fields, cleaners, polishes, disinfectants, insect repellants, household pesticides, medications, beauty products (both cleansing and cosmetic), toilet paper, food and cookware, bedding, clothing, other textiles, office and art supplies, home finishing products, infant and toddler toys, and pet products. *Home Safe Home* has a wealth of information regarding products not normally known to be toxic, as well as telling why each item is toxic. Basically, if a product is not marketed as all-natural (and you should still read the ingredients), you can be assured that the product was conventionally produced and full of chemicals which *are* harmful in one way or another to the human body. There are many unavoidable pollutants, as well as products for which no natural alternatives are made, and it is wise to be apprised of the risks. Acquire *Home Safe Home* and similar books to find out more about chemical pollutants.

You may ask whether there is really a cause for concern. Study after study is realizing the consequences of poor choices. I can only imagine where we will be thirty years from now if these trends escalate. The fact that mankind *doesn't know everything about everything* should induce caution. While something appears harmless now, there may very likely be some aspect unknown to us that will end up causing great harm. Unquestionably, this has been the case with manmade chemicals. Using natural products is always best because *God does know everything* and He created plants, animals, and minerals specifically for our resources.

The "instincts, upbringing, and personal tastes" mentioned below are mainly products of the last couple of generations—decades which have been saturated by modern popular culture. We *must* have a larger scope and assess the changes that are happening due to unprecedented leaps in manufacturing, information technology, and disease rates.

We are grappling with a new problem here, for which there is no precedent. We have reached the point at which we must be informed consumers—we can no longer rely on our instincts, upbringing, personal tastes, or what is easily available in stores to guide us as we shop. We must learn the risks and how to minimize them. If we ignore the toxic problems in our world, they won't go away—they will only get worse.[12]

In a Google search I performed about "man-made chemicals," I found the headlines below, which are only a sampling of what appeared. Due to previous research, these were not surprising.

- Man-made chemicals detected in newborns
- Man-made chemicals reduce animals' masculinity
- Male alligators born in this lake contaminated by manmade chemicals are showing dramatic changes in their reproductive systems
- Man-made chemicals have the ability to mimic hormones
- Man-made chemicals found in baby fat, breast milk, and terrestrial and aquatic life
- Man-made chemicals are severely undermining the reproductive health of wildlife and humans the world over
- Man-made chemicals in maternal and umbilical cord blood
- Man-made chemicals found in drinking water
- Risks from man-made chemicals are increasingly putting women and children in danger

As a side note, many Christian leaders today are beginning to teach about biblical male and female roles and are lamenting the growing prevalence of lessened masculinity and femininity in our country. I would submit that one reason for this dearth of proper roles is that hormones are being chemically disrupted. It is not only a lack of fearing God and a lack of proper training that leads to ignorance and disobedience of biblical roles, but also the presence of deficient, even harmful, diets. Though there is no substitute for godly instruction, we need to be careful of how altered foods and manmade chemicals can unknowingly compromise our optimal condition. Manmade chemicals attack God's orderly universe in more ways than one: they pollute the earth and they mess with humankind.

Not only chemicals, but crops like soy, can change hormones. Though soy was even recently claimed as a health food, most of the nutritionists whose work I have studied have detected major faults with soy and warn against its use. Soy naturally contains high concentrations of female hormones and is being used in everything from cattle feed, to oils in baked goods, to soy flour and soy protein in practically every food product on the market. People complain that girls are physically maturing at younger ages and that boys are becoming more effeminate. We need to study and rethink every aspect of our diets, especially relatively recent products such as man-made chemical additives or processed soy products, the usage of which has greatly increased in the last few decades.

Chemicals are foreign to our bodies and that fact alone is enough to induce caution, even if neither you nor I understand exactly how or why chemicals harm us. Though anyone can notice trends, the Christian's task is to be vigilant for holy living in the wicked world we live in. My hope is that my readers become convinced and concerned that we must unconditionally live our lives in a way that honors God's purposes for the earth and for our bodies.

The simple truth is, what protects the earth also protects our bodies, and what harms the earth also harms our bodies. For instance, pesticides are good neither for accumulation in the earth's soil and water, or for buildup in our blood and organs. The actions that most acknowledge His perfect creating power in the earth are the same actions that most nourish the delicate anatomy of our human bodies and our capability to bring other God-fearing generations into the world. Natural food and natural household products benefit everyone at every level.

Dr. Colbert prompts the reader to action. Don't we all want to live in a healthy home? Then we need to purposefully and methodically *reclaim* its environment, as he suggests, and design a refuge from the inevitable perils outside.

> A safe, healthy home is a gift and a powerful haven of blessed refuge from the battles of daily life. To consider that, without your knowing it, poisonous, cancer-causing substances have been polluting that haven and attacking you and your family is offensive...Armed with knowledge and practical advice, you can reclaim the healthful environment of your home.[13]

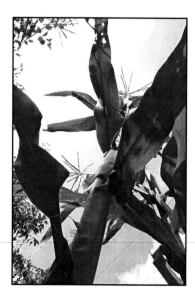

Chapter Fifteen

The Plague of Regulations

"If people let government dictate what foods they eat and what medicines they take, their bodies will soon be in as sorry a state as are the souls of those who live under tyranny."[1]
—Thomas Jefferson

AROUND THE THIRTEENTH century, "sophistication" was the term used for adding a foreign or inferior substance to food; sophistication was punishable by a humiliating sentence in the pillory. Refined sugar, a brand new commodity in the Western world, was one such substance understood to have the effects of "sophistication" in products to which it was added, especially in alcohol. The effects of small amounts of sugar in people's diets caused such strange and previously unknown symptoms that state and church leaders accused the presence of abnormal behavior on bewitchment. Natural healers who knew the real cause of the behavior and blamed it on sugar could be condemned as wizards and burned at the stake for their opinions.

In the present day, Western Civilization is sophisticated in its own way. The causes of problems are not discussed. Living in this civilization, we tend to ignore the truth of how anything is processed. We treat symptoms with drugs instead of changing the addicting diets we have grown to love. Instead of being punished for altering food as in medieval times, we act like the food is fine. One thing has not changed though: natural methods of healing—methods that resist the powers-that-be—are heavily censored.

111

God has always tended to work through minority numbers of people, even in the realm of science. Perseverance is often eventually rewarded, but then new controversies appear on the scene, forming a perpetual pattern:

> The history of science is the history of struggle against entrenched error. Many of the world's greatest discoveries initially were rejected by the scientific community. And those who pioneered those discoveries often were ridiculed and condemned as quacks or charlatans.[2]

Practitioners that supply supplements and natural remedies are not allowed to state any healing benefits. Raw milk is not legal for sale in most of the United States. While naturopaths and other alternative physicians are allowed to practice, they are seldom given any credit by the mass media or bureaucratic officeholders. These natural practitioners know how cancer forms, for instance, and know many things that can prevent it, yet they are hushed while the American Cancer Society labors away, getting funding from pharmaceutical corporations and making money from treating cancer, while ignoring and discriminating against organizations that have discovered alternative treatments. With little accountability from the bottom-up, our nation in general is ignorant of the issues at stake and is wasting away in the process.

The treatment of cancer with vitamin B_{17}, also known as laetrile, is one example. The FDA does not allow health claims to be made along with the marketing of B_{17}. Hence, various laetrile therapy institutes exist, but they are outside of the United States in other North American and European countries. G. Edward Griffin, who wrote *World Without Cancer*, speaks forcefully to this issue. His boldness is to be applauded:

> Each year, thousands of Americans travel to Mexico and Germany to receive Laetrile therapy. They do this because it has been suppressed in the United States. Most of these patients have been told their cancer is terminal and they have but a few months to live. Yet, an incredible percentage of them have recovered and are living normal lives. However, the FDA, the AMA, the American Cancer Society, and the cancer research centers continue to pronounce that Laetrile is quackery...

> If any of these patients ultimately die after seeking Laetrile, spokesmen for orthodox medicine are quick to proclaim: 'You see? Laetrile doesn't work!' Meanwhile, hundreds of thousands of patients die each year after undergoing surgery, radiation, or chemotherapy, but those treatments continue to be touted as 'safe and effective.'[3]

National medical organizations and federal health and agriculture departments do not give much credence to preventative measures. The views of the people in controlling positions are that problems can be resolved from the top-down and from the outside-in. Their regulations, their lobbying, their campaigns, and their money always go to support the philosophy that human wisdom can fix human problems using human methods. Unless men fear God, regulations and influence will always be weighted toward the allowance of more chemical additives, the forced use of vaccines and drugs, the scorn of dietary nutrition, and the stifling of non-invasive procedures such as chiropractic, homeopathic, or natural supplementation. People who do not fear God are working against His purposes, and in the end, His purposes are the only ones that will stand. We are repeatedly reminded of this in the Psalms and Proverbs.

> The labour of the righteous tendeth to life: the fruit of the wicked to sin...The fear of the LORD prolongeth days: but the years of the wicked shall be shortened. The hope of the righteous shall be gladness: but the expectation of the wicked shall perish. The way of the LORD is strength to the upright: but destruction shall be to the workers of iniquity. The righteous shall never be removed: but the wicked shall not inhabit the earth.
>
> —Proverbs 10:16, 27–30

Government-marketed health advice, such as the USDA (United States Department of Agriculture) food pyramid, is widely thought by consumers to be a basic standard for diet, but it is very flawed. Forty percent of our calories should come from good fats, yet the food pyramid lumps fats and sweets together as if they are equally to be avoided. We would thrive with no refined sugars, yet we are in distinct need of the proper quantity of healthy fats and oils. Some of the foods at the base of the pyramid (cereal, crackers, etc.) have a higher glycemic index (creating more blood sugar) than straight sugar does, and yet we are supposed to make processed grains a full fifty-five percent of our diet! The rise in obesity, diabetes, heart disease, and cancer is due in large part to the food industry's impact on, and consumer following of, the USDA food guidelines. As the next quotation supports, the *quality* of the fats, carbohydrates, and proteins that we eat is much more important than the volume, proportions, or number of calories received.

Below, Sally Fallon Morell offers a penetrating critique of modern national guidelines. The USDA Food Pyramid is based more on what food looks like and the dollars it brings in, than on what food is made of and the nutrients it brings into the body. With the commercial food industry's regard for current profit more than for the time-honored standards of history, this is hardly surprising. (Seeing the flaws with the USDA Pyramid, other organizations have created whole-food, Mediterranean, or vegetarian pyramids for better guidelines.) Isn't the following critique incisive? It definitely draws "a line in the sand":

The new [USDA Food Pyramid] guidelines perpetuate the myth that fats, carbohydrates and proteins have equal nutritional properties no matter how much or how little they are processed. The experts make no distinction between whole grains and refined, between foods grown organically and those grown with pesticides and commercial fertilizers, between unprocessed dairy products from pasture-fed cows and pasteurized dairy products from confined animals raised on processed feed, between fresh and rancid fats, between traditional fresh fruits and vegetables and those that have been irradiated or genetically altered, between range-fed meats and those from animals raised in crowded pens, between natural and battery-produced eggs; in short, between the traditional foods that nourished our ancestors and newfangled products now dominating the modern marketplace.[4]

My premise thus far has been that Christians need to give thought to the food we eat, indeed, to be as knowledgeable as we can about it. This premise suggests that we need to do the research ourselves, not relying on umbrella agencies such as the Food and Drug Administration (FDA) or commercial food producers' associations to protect our health. Organizations do serve their place, I suppose, insofar as they establish production, transportation, and marketing standards for one of the largest industries in the world. However, there are several issues of concern with the FDA. One issue is that countless chemicals are approved as additives, as preservatives, and as part of manufacturing processes—chemicals that are quite harmful as they accumulate in the body. Another issue is that the FDA regulates and inhibits the health claims and distribution of natural food and natural remedies.

When food is intended to last longer and be transported farther, the amount of additives increases. Additives change food so that it does not do what it normally does: nourish you if it is eaten and deteriorate if it is not eaten. With current manufacturing techniques, processed food does less of both: it lasts a very long time, and it nourishes you very little. The farther the FDA gets from pure, simple food, the less we can trust them. How can this much regulation exist at the government level without bureaucrats getting carried away with their influence over food, drugs, and their attempt to oversee everything in the nation? I contest that "there is no fear of God before their eyes" in their love of money, their use of power, or their concern for human health.

Financially interconnected, it is difficult for either the food industry, medical industry, universities, or government agencies to be completely objective in their interests. As seen in the following quotation, the food industry is probably the most dominant of the four entities I just mentioned.

The Diet Dictocrats are strangely silent about the ever increasing trend toward food processing and the devitalization of America's rich agricultural bounty. Food processing is the largest manufacturing industry in the country and hence the most powerful. This industry naturally uses its financial clout to influence the slant of university research and the dictates that come from government agencies.[5]

Food is *not* a neutral issue; the FDA does not have a high respect for God's creation of the environment or of our bodies. The FDA approves many harmful ingredients because it neither wants nor tries to know what the long-term effects are and it does not regard long-term effects as much as Christians should. As thoughtful Christians commanded to be distinct from the world, we do not accept everything that the world does in behavior, music, art, relationships, or anything else. We need to think differently than the world, the government, and our sin nature. We need to think God's thoughts after Him—as the great scientist Johann Kepler proposed and demonstrated—and seek to do things, even eating, in His way. If we keep thinking human thoughts after the way of mankind, we will be led further in the wrong direction—away from God our Creator, Sustainer, and Redeemer.

Harmful substances are constantly being approved with no basis for their environmental or consumption safety. Every time I do research, I read another article on a study conducted by medical doctors or medical laboratories (usually in the United Kingdom or Australia, it seems) that shows a correlation between a certain drug or substance and a certain behavior or disease. Recently, I have read that nitrates are a cause of sudden infant death syndrome; that vaccinations are a cause of autism; and that the drug Ritalin™ has been known to cause depression and schizophrenia. Limitless information, too broad to list here, can be gathered about the dangers of artificial and chemical substances. Please be advised to always approach modern developments with the intent to research them. Conduct research thoroughly (meaning not only from the viewpoint of the person recommending it) before consenting to ingest a food or medicine.

Another issue regarding the FDA is that this organization would not be necessary if we purchased food locally from trustworthy growers—growers who are willing to show and personally tell you how they operate. The food is fresh; consumers know about their food; the free market helps good producers to prosper; and the need for top-down control from the government is eliminated. The FDA serves its position because of a vicious cycle in our society. If we are far from the origins of our food, standards are somewhat comforting. If we see grocery store aisles more than we see farmers' fields, nationally-certified claims of quality are the best assurance we can have.

Large food businesses use their fortunes to lobby marketing associations and Congress, who, in turn, makes laws that favor the commercialized food industry. Many former corporate officers of giant food corporations now hold federal offices and are supposed to be regulating the very companies that have made their fortune. Current laws are favoring the centralization of large food companies while discriminating against decentralization of agriculture, including entrepreneurship of small businesses. The media goes along with the same sentiments that are advertised by food companies and promoted by Congress. Lately, numerous articles easily discounted as false have claimed that fast food is good for you, that sugar is harmless, that cell phones are safe, and that artificial products have no known side effects. Profitable food manufacturing is not wrong in the least. However, ultimate greed for money and power will lead to more corruption at every level.

Healthcare seemed to be the major concern on the minds of many during the recent U.S. Presidential election of 2008. American health is failing and medical care is costing more than ever before. Our nation is aging and is staggered by disease. Topics of discussion centered on *how much* spending was necessary and on *where* to put the money, not whether all the programs and agencies are constitutional or helpful in the first place. The primary variable debated was the *extent* of the government's help. Disturbingly, the scheme of nationalizing the medical industry arose.

While all of the other candidates before and after the primaries seemed to stake all their trust in government departments and the pharmaceutical industry, Presidential candidate Dr. Ron Paul was the opposite. He believes in *health freedom*—in the idea that people should be able to know the truth about nutritional supplements without these being monopolized and suppressed by "Big Pharma." Congressman Dr. Ron Paul from Texas has been the most outspoken voice for health freedom in Congress recently; numerous times, he has introduced the Health Freedom Protection Act which would give back freedom of speech to nutritional companies. The Act would have allowed for claims to be made about the nutrition and health benefits of food products. Currently, the FDA enforces a "prior restraint" such that benefits have to be proven before they can be claimed. In his words on the House floor, Dr. Paul explained the facts behind his actions:

> Because of the FDA's censorship of truthful health claims, millions of Americans may suffer with diseases and other health care problems they may have avoided by using dietary supplements....Specifically, the Health Freedom Protection Act stops the FDA from censoring truthful claims about the curative, mitigative, or preventative effects of dietary supplements, and adopts the federal court's suggested use of disclaimers as an alternative to censorship. The Health Freedom Protection Act also stops the FDA from prohibiting the distribution of scientific articles and publications regarding the role of nutrients in protecting against disease.[6]

The bottom line is that the United States government cannot protect our health even if doing so were its responsibility. Health is the responsibility of each person to attend to on their own. It is the responsibility of citizens to be aware of the measures that Congress and the FDA are effecting and to elect wise men to national offices. Once a government becomes this enlarged, money and power begin to be more attractive than the good of the nation. Indeed, our government is too large to be either prudent or efficient in the management of medicine and agriculture. The FDA will not admit that nutrition prevents disease; therefore, nutrition companies are so hushed from giving health advice that an entire sector of the market is made quite vulnerable to FDA control instead of being captive to the truth.

If we do not make choices now—both in the people we elect and in the foods we select—there may come a day when the government controls choices even more closely. The author of one online article, after mentioning the whole foods that we should choose and the processed foods that we should avoid, gives the following warning:

> However, if we, the people, allow the government too much control over agriculture and the food industry, we may not have much of a choice in what is available to us in the future. As always, be educated, be aware, and be involved.[7]

At the risk of giving examples that will sound outdated, the United States Congress has recently considered measures for requiring various vaccines; mandating specific drugs for women, girls, and boys; and forcing input and licensing output of the smallest farms and roadside stands. The same drugs and chemicals that the FDA allows are the same things that Congress will seek to make universal. Many of the measures that U.S. government agencies are taking are every bit as injurious as the terrorist activities in foreign countries.

Many Americans, even those who are politically conservative, tend to speak of the rest of the world's problems rather than addressing our own. If we would pay more attention to our own government, we would know what was really going on behind the guise of science. Notice the author's use of the word "sophistication" here—the concept with which this chapter began:

> Terrorists are not just 'them,' they are 'us.' Western terrorists are more sophisticated. Our domestic terrorists do not blow up schoolhouses, they splice genes. They destroy healthy cows in the name of science. They give chemical companies free roads and dump sights [sic]. They feed brains and spinal cords to cows. They lock up pigs and chickens in concentration camps—and feed the adulterated carcasses to our nation's school children.[8]

Advocacy of health freedom in the last election was more than timely, as it came alongside a new inspiration for multitudes of Americans to cherish and protect liberty. Continued interest in this issue is important at every level for the sake of our individual lives as well as the liberty of our nation. A government that does not fear God will continue trying to act like a god in its grasp for power, and will continue traveling down a path that leads toward sin, injustice, and destruction. As Christians begin to make changes in their health habits at the personal level, they need to be aware of, and willing to take action in, the area of health freedom.

G. Edward Griffin speaks specifically about cancer in this quotation, but his thoughts are broadly relevant. His perceptiveness about both bureaucracy leadership and grass-roots opposition is rare:

> Already there is a growing backlash at the grass-roots level. With thousands of cancer victims providing living testimony to the effectiveness of vitamin B_{17}, with hundreds of thousands discovering the value of nutrition, in spite of FDA-AMA pronouncements to the contrary, with Watergate and Whitewater scandals leading millions to realize that they neither can believe nor trust their political leaders, we are coming to a point of open resistance to government which could make the Boston Tea Party look like child's play.[9]

The government's trying to regulate healthcare from the top-down is nothing new. Three and a half centuries ago, around the time of the English Civil War and the Protectorate of Oliver Cromwell, an apothecary and naturalist was able to challenge what was basically state control over the manufacture and prescription of natural remedies. Nicholas Culpeper challenged the London College of Physicians by getting knowledge to the common person. Like the English were in the seventeenth century, America today is separated from her roots. We have been ignorant of history; we do not inform ourselves about the government's meddling in concerns of individual health or in medicinal treatments. We often do not know what is in food or drugs, and we suffer the government to decide what is best.

British author Benjamin Woolley documents the life of apothecary Nicholas Culpeper in his compelling biography *Heal Thyself: Nicholas Culpeper and the Seventeenth Century Struggle to Bring Medicine to the People.* His book is of relevance in a time when our current American government has similar aspirations as the College of Physicians and a time when people should take courage to do what they know is right, including the disseminating of information.

Christians are eternally thankful, of course, that men were courageous to translate, print, and distribute the Bible in the sixteenth century when it was more than frowned upon. Likewise, any dissemination of truth should be a worthy cause. Nicholas Culpeper spread truth to the Society of Apothecaries and the English people; Mr. Woolley revives and retells his story for people to understand today. The attractive writing style in *Heal Thyself* seems to bring the reader right back into the medical and power struggles of old London.

No apothecary should be allowed to make any medicine without a 'living Doctor's bill', he [William Harvey of the College of Physicians] said. Furthermore, they should take an oath to make only those medicines set out in the official *Pharmacopoeia Londinensis* (to prevent them selling compounds of their own) which should be sold by prices fixed by the College...It was a devastating attack, and provoked a furious response from the Society of Apothecaries, targeted directly at Harvey.[10]

Despite the popularity of medicines such as London Treacle, the *Pharmacopoeia* gave no hint as to their medicinal qualities. This was to confine the apothecaries to preparing medicines and to prevent them from prescribing them.[11]

Nicholas Culpeper saw the need for the humble apothecary, and also the common person, to have the knowledge of what they were producing (in the apothecary's case) and what they were procuring (in the patient's case.) He regarded the knowledge of men more than the control of the elite. Great repercussions ensued as both parties reacted to this novel upheaval in the medical system. The American colonies, starting out with more respect for liberty than for royalty, evidently favored the individual acquisition of knowledge above dependence upon a governing body of physicians.

By writing the *English Physitian* or *Herbal* he established the principle of the public right to know. He made medical knowledge widely accessible to ordinary people for the first time, and their appetite proved to be inexhaustible...It became one of the most popular books in colonial America where many of Nicholas' Puritan brethren probably appreciated its political message as much as its medical one. As late as 1770, doctors in Boston, Massachusetts, tried to set up a college of Physicians of their own, but found their efforts frustrated by the conviction among 'every plain honest country gentleman and judicious citizen that reading Culpeper's *English Physician enlarged*' provided them with all the medical knowledge they needed.[12]

In his 1647 translation of the *Pharmacopoeia*, Nicholas Culpeper gave English recipes for all the remedies that apothecaries made and told the apothecaries and the common people what curative effects the remedies had. Mr. Woolley says that this promoted "community values versus commercial interests" and "simple natural remedies versus complex artificial compounds."[13] In the front of his new edition, Culpeper wrote a rather strong political statement, but one that has often been true in the history of the world.

...the Liberty of our Common-Wealth (if I may call it so without a Solecism) is most infringed by three sorts of men, Priests, Physicians, Lawyers. The one deceives men in matters belonging to their Souls, the other in matters belonging to their Bodies, the third in matters belonging to their Estates.[14]

In the medical and religious freedoms of individuals, America originally contradicted the sentiments in the previous quotation. However, the common person in our country is now, again, nearly as ignorant as English citizens were before Culpeper's edition of the *Pharmacopoeia*. Americans don't often know what is in the "compounds" used, and we trust physicians and "royal societies" to safeguard our health.

The times were changing in seventeenth-century Britain, and industries and trades were no longer so closely guarded by the aristocracy or governed by professionals. While Americans still hold on to the statement from our Declaration of Independence that "all men are created equal," more of a class system exists than we would like to admit. The bureaucracy wants to perform things without the citizens' knowledge and does not want the people to perform their own measures—such as private regulation of small farms wherein the free market would regulate itself. America does need to return to the sentiments of the colonial-era patriots—ideologically as well as practically.

In his thought-provoking Epilogue, author Benjamin Woolley describes the influence of the English apothecary and the timeliness of Culpeper's beliefs for the present. This perspective is very interesting and is worth considering.

> What Culpeper did was challenge the principle that medical knowledge belonged solely to physicians—indeed that expert knowledge of any sort belonged to the experts. He helped to reveal a division that has yet to heal, between orthodox and alternative medicine, between professional expertise and personal empowerment.[15]

In the American Revolution, one hundred and thirty years after the time of Culpeper and presently two hundred and thirty years in the past, the concern for a free commonwealth was again boldly addressed. The Founding Fathers sought to ensure "life, liberty, and the pursuit of happiness" by the establishing of checks and balances, the respect for institutional jurisdictions, and the protection of private property.

Local, decentralized control is a principle of biblical government, church, and family. Local control can apply also to health when individual families and individual states take responsibility for making their own decisions rather than voting for health decisions to be made by the federal government. In the area of health and nutrition, we need to be aware of changes happening at the top—from the federal government, in order to counteract these changes from the bottom—through families, private businesses, and individual states.

Chapter Sixteen

Buying What We Believe

"Money is not the only capital of agriculture. Rivers, streams, forests, soil, air, water—they all belong to our natural capital."[1]

—Steve Meyerowitz

CONSUMERS OF GOODS and services are not mindless disposers but are creators, in a sense, and voters.[2] We shape not only our own lifestyles by what we buy, but also the disposition of the selling market. The use of our pocketbooks is a powerful technique for promoting the things we believe in. We cannot complain about the carelessness of the large commercialized food industry and simultaneously complain about the high prices or low availability of natural foods. With our monies, we can show that we do not appreciate the mega-food industry and do appreciate conscientious farmers and businesses.

Where possible, Christians should give their money to businesses with integrity in marketing—whose advertising tells the truth about the origin of the product rather than making groundless claims about people's happiness after eating it! Supporting companies that work for the highest excellence of culinary quality is a good endeavor, as opposed to supporting companies that churn out the cheapest, fastest food products imaginable. We need to make a practice of purchasing organic or natural products if we want to nourish ourselves and help the earth stay cleaner.

Christians should do as much as possible to support businesses that seek to follow God's principles of stewardship over the earth and our bodies. Some of our tax money already goes to subsidize massive food corporations, while small businesses are hurting under the tax burden and oppressive laws. (Besides, the subsidies are largely going toward the manufacture of commodity crops wheat, corn, and soy—foods that become ultra cheap to the consumer and therefore comprise much of the unhealthful American diet.) While we can never control the very last place that our dollar goes and whether it supports anything against our beliefs, purchasing from local agriculture markets and small organic companies is a great place to start.

Costs can fool us, explains Steve Meyerowitz in *The Organic Food Guide*. Behind the price on the can, there are many costs and processes that ultimately affect our pocketbooks:

> For many years our society was convinced that cheaper food was better. But such is no longer the case. The residual costs of chemicals in agriculture are coming back to haunt us in the form of polluted air, water, and food—and ultimately higher taxes for the cost of cleanup and the effects on public health. Unfortunately, it has taken us a few decades to learn that the cost of using chemicals in agriculture is more than just the [comparatively lower] price on the can.[3]

"I have rejoiced in the way of thy testimonies, as much as in all riches," reads Psalm 119:14. As this verse indicates, honoring God's Word and His revelation about His creation is more important, I think, than hoarding our money and not being willing to spend it on wholesome food. The "way of His testimonies" is what Christians should rejoice in, though most people rejoice in their riches. Are we more concerned about the thriftiest bargains on food, or about pleasing God with wise purchases? Though Isaiah 55:2 is speaking of spiritual sustenance, this verse asks a good question which can be applied to our daily bread: "Wherefore do ye spend money for that which is not bread? and your labour for that which satisfieth not? hearken diligently unto me, and eat ye that which is good." Are we more concerned with the quantity of our money than with the quality of products that our money buys? This should not be. Additionally, some people think they are saving money on food, but what they are buying is hardly real food and does not provide real nourishment.

One common complaint is that organic and natural food can be much more expensive. As you know, Americans judge the quality and longevity of everything we purchase. For instance, we always try to buy as much vehicle as we can with an allotted amount of money. We only buy something old and prone to breakage if that is all we can afford, with full knowledge of its limitations and its propensity to cause us difficulty and more expense. If we are insistent upon reliability in a vehicle, we will get a newer one and pay the higher price for the sake of traveling ease. The case is similar with food.

Better quality foods tend to cost more. We have to decide whether the extra money spent on good food is a worthy investment in our health, just as we decide how much money we are willing to forego for the sake of safe and comfortable transportation. (Conversely, processed food that costs more than unprocessed food is not a gauge of quality; cost of technology is the issue there, where price is an indicator of convenience rather than of nutritional value.) We always prioritize what we are willing to spend money on. For instance, diminishing one's spending on high-cost processed convenience foods, restaurant meals, and less-than-necessary goods, services, or recreation can help pay for the cost of organic, natural food.

Possibly, we should perceive conventional food as costing *less*, not organic food as costing *more*. If conventional food has filler ingredients—not real food—we're not only paying for food, we're also paying for things that are *not* food. The prices have been dropped because the processes are becoming inferior; denatured food begs a lower price. The price of good quality food, then, should be our standard. We should realize that conventional food costs *less* than food should cost and that, by paying *more*, we're purchasing the real thing.

How often do we buy the cheapest or least expensive choices of a given product? We always define the standard at some point. Buying the least expensive version of a good quality item is understandable, but there are not many products in which we willingly forego quality altogether. If we had, we would all be living in rags and shacks. Assuming we have money in our purses, by God's grace, we are always choosing what to save it for and what to spend it on. Since we are always making judgments in regard to quality, our standard for food needs to be raised from low quality to a much higher quality of excellence as well as nutritional value. While raising our standard, we will be supporting businesses who try hard to provide wholesome, quality products. The wonderful news is that, due to technology and entrepreneurialism, healthier alternatives for just about every food are widely available. Most of all, we need to be informed if we are going to make wise decisions.

Much more than personal health is benefited by organic purchases. One benefit is the health of our neighbors "downstream and downwind," as Michael Pollan writes. I would add—caring for our neighbors is a Christian duty, is it not?

> There's no escaping the fact that better food—whether measured by taste or nutritional quality (which often correspond) –costs more, usually because it has been grown with more care and less intensively... [Buying better food] benefits not only your health (by, among other things, reducing your exposure to pesticides and pharmaceuticals), but also the health of the people who grow the food as well as the people who live downstream and downwind of the farms where it is grown. Another important benefit of paying more for better-quality food is that you're apt to eat less of it.[4]

While organic food will typically cost more than non-organic food, there is no reason why eating wholesome natural foods would ever be more expensive than eating refined and processed foods. Ready-to-eat or precooked foods often cost from four to ten times more than the cost of single, unprepared foods such as raw meat or raw potatoes. Wholesome, homemade food is usually less expensive (for the volume and for the nourishment) than processed food or restaurant meals, though organic ingredients are more expensive than their conventionally-grown counterparts. For this reason, many people I know don't buy every single ingredient in its certified-organic version, but they do buy everything as wholesome, natural, and as local as possible. Besides, natural food nourishes you better, so you can eat less of it.

Since the resources used in the mass-producing of refined conventional foods are grown cheaply and with low quality, prices have to be high not mainly to cover the price of the ingredients, but to pay for the latest processing technology and all the steps and hands involved. You support industrialism, poor health, and low-quality, high-impact agricultural practices if you buy this food. Since the resources used in the niche-producing of wholesome organic foods take special care and attention, the profit counted into their prices pays mostly for the time and initial cost of more expensive resources. You support low-impact, high-quality agricultural practices and better health if you buy this food. Farming—husbandry of the land—is a noble vocation when it is done well, and is a heritage worth protecting.

The above contrast is provided not to say there are only two types of production, which there are not, but only to show where the emphasis for profit is with companies who pursue magnitude of production versus companies that pursue superiority of product. The policies which our dollar empowers are a matter of money versus health, and of efficiency versus quality.

What are the benefits of money moving between local businesses? Mr. Meyerowitz answers. The preference should be obvious between beautiful communities versus factory farms than ruin ecosystems.

> Agricultural policies today favor factory farms, giant supermarkets, and long-distance trade. But if we were to spend our money on locally-grown foods, these dollars would likely stay in the region, create jobs, and buy local goods and services. Small organic and local farms help the environment and preserve the character and beauty of a community.[5]

Since what is paid for with convenience foods is the machinery and time for processing and packaging, it is economically prudent to do more processing in your home, which will be necessary if you buy whole, unprepared foods. If you use your own time to prepare foods for consumption—whether for that evening's meal, for tomorrow's picnic, or for winter sustenance—you cut down on expenditure, avoid industrialization, and connect with and learn more about your meal in the process.[6] When we spend time making and enjoying our food, we are apt to appreciate it more than if it we just grabbed it off of a shelf and quickly consumed it from a package. When we don't need to spend time preparing food that technology has already prepared, we are apt to eat more of it than we should, as one author believes.[7] Though processed food costs more money, it does not cost much time, and people often appreciate the time saved in buying and eating already-prepared foods. However, if we want to save money, we will have to spend time on food preparation.

In her cookbook *Hearth and Home*, Karey Swan gives some practical tips about home cooking. The percentage of savings that she cites is intriguing. If this percentage is still accurate, no one has a reason to complain about replacing convenience foods with organic foods.

Well, serious cooking requires knowledge of basic physics and chemistry, as well as nutrition. Knowing your ingredients and the importance of freshness and quality combined with culinary skills and proper training in the use of kitchen tools, brings cooking to the level of craft or art...

Cooking from scratch is simply putting a recipe together using whole, fresh food rather than purchasing processed food. It is grinding your own flour, mixing it with baking powder, eggs, and milk instead of using a purchased pancake mix. It is making your own soup stock and cutting up fresh vegetables instead of reaching for canned soup...

The higher nutritional value and lower cost of cooking from scratch is substantial, not to mention the superior taste. The average family would cut 30% to 50% off their grocery bill and at the same time improve their health by cooking from scratch. With the availability of bulk whole food we enjoy today, kitchen machines that do most of the work, and the mountain of how-to books, cooking from scratch is within the reach of virtually every family.[8]

Buying ingredients in bulk and cooking from scratch with them is the most healthful way to prepare meals. Buying fresh produce in the summertime, hunting for wild meat or purchasing a side of beef in the fall, and storing grain from that season's harvest are good ways to know from where your food has come. People historically had to eat with the seasons—eating garden food in the summer and preserved food in the winter (canned, frozen, or dehydrated food.) When consumers of late have desired fresh food in every season, farmers have had to imitate the seasons in greenhouses (for plants) and factories (for animals), or else food is flown in from tropical climates.[9] Not only do those measures heighten costs, but the nutritional quality of food is low if it has been grown with artificial light or stored for long periods of time. Have you ever had pale, expensive strawberries or tomatoes off-season? They are underdeveloped in comparison to the bright, juicy, fruit picked from a garden in the summer or frozen or canned for the winter.

Most of what my family buys comes under one of the following categories: 1) locally or regionally grown or distributed by companies with which we are familiar; or 2) organic or all-natural, and certified by a third party organization with high standards. We search out the ingredients no matter where the food or product comes from, especially if it was not locally grown or certified organic. We try to buy from an all-natural wholesale delivery company when possible[10] as well as buying direct from producers at their businesses or at farmers' markets during the summer.

You can do it! Use the medium of commerce—markets, cooperatives, small businesses, and grocery stores—to your advantage and for the promotion of the principles discussed. Do not view chain stores as the sole and unquestioned source of your every need, but go to wherever quality is found. *In Defense of Food* here defends the best sources of food:

> The surest way to escape the Western diet is simply to depart the realm it rules: the supermarket, the convenience store, and the fast food outlet. It is hard to eat badly from the farmers' market, from a CSA box (community-supported agriculture, an increasingly popular scheme in which you subscribe to a farm and receive a weekly box of produce), or from your garden.[11]

The "realm it rules"—a fitting depiction from Michael Pollan about the food industry. To what realm will you, the reader, subject your dollars, your food, and ultimately your body? It should be a realm where more noble principles are at work, I hope, since we are citizens of Christ's kingdom! It should be a realm where food is seen as a tool to be treasured more than a commodity to be churned out. Fortunately, there is such a possibility.

For whole foods, my family leans toward the side of regionally-grown foods. For instance, when we don't make our own bread, we buy it from a local bakery. When we do make bread, we use grain from a local grower. Local foods are typically produced in small volume, and since more can be known about their production, choosing local foods is the closest thing to growing food or preparing it at home. For prepared foods (ready to eat from a box, bottle, or bag), my family leans toward the side of organically-produced foods. When we buy condiments or snacks, we try to get those with the most natural ingredients. Wide varieties of prepared foods are not usually manufactured in regions of small population such as our state, but by purchasing from organic companies when we cannot buy locally, we still support good standards of agriculture and production.

Basically no organic household products, such as laundry detergent or hair conditioner, are manufactured in our region, so I make sure to buy those from organic companies that distribute to local natural food markets.

We should buy as much regionally-produced and conscientiously-produced food as possible in order to facilitate knowledge of the product we are buying and encourage localized control of the food industry. There is no reason we should be eating apples from the Orient—hardly a regional purchase, not to mention our knowing nothing about the growth of the apple—when apples are grown in basically every region in the United States. While we may wish we could change health and nutrition practices from the top-down, change will not happen that way. Most worthwhile endeavors are accomplished from the bottom-up by small steps of faithful people. We can make responsible choices for ourselves, and the more that Christian families begin to make wise choices, the bigger difference it will make in the food market.

Joel Salatin, a farmer whom I have quoted several times and a writer who has done much to help others replicate his farming philosophy, has more faith in local food than in organic food. His point, which is well-taken, is that organic cooperatives are being bought up by Wall Street companies and that organic standards will be compromised as a result. He says that ninety-five percent of organic foods in health food stores come from just as far away as their conventional counterparts, and that we know hardly any more about the way organic foods are processed.[12] Personal inspection of, or inquiry about, a farmer's agricultural practices will always leave a customer with more knowledge than would trusting the USDA Organic certification.

However, if organic subsidiaries, even of Wall Street companies, are maintaining their organic certification, I would put more faith in the organic version than in the conventional version of a product that I cannot acquire locally. The fact that huge corporations are willing to buy organic companies does show, encouragingly, how exponentially the organic market is growing and is expected to grow. Large companies might be changing the nature of organic companies to some extent when the latter are acquired; yet, organic companies are in turn becoming a larger, more influential part of the wider market. With a caveat for when buying certified organic is the only option, the wisest choice is still to be more connected with your food—to know more about it—by buying it from farmers you trust.

In our culture, as Joel Salatin believes, we subject many professions to scrutiny before we use their services—but the farmers who grow our food are often left unnoticed. We like to personally interview a babysitter, for instance—and with good reason—but when it comes to eating, we tend to trust everything said and made by the industrial food system.[13] He suggests an alternative to fragmentation and calls this connectedness:

If I were to choose one word to summarize the kind of food buyers who patronize farm friendly fare, it would have to be 'connected.' All of us have to work at being connected because fragmentation is the easiest thing in the world.[14]

What could possibly be more important to our family, our children, our grandchildren, our community, our world, than getting connected to our food system? Are we wanting to just rant and rave about multinational control? Would we rather scowl at untrustworthy food giants who seem to be recalling food at least once a week?[15]

While some people go shopping to look for the most exotic imports or the cheapest bargains or their favorite snacks, we need to go looking for the healthiest foods. Local or organic naturally-raised and thoughtfully-produced foods are treasures to be sought if we would only make the effort. They reward the consumer not only with superb taste but with a satisfied assurance of well-being for eating wholesomely and supporting good motives.

As anything grows, it matures, and so has the organic food movement over the last fifty years leading up to the present. In *The Organic Food Guide*, a great resource for any consumer, Steve Meyerowitz has some helpful commentary. He emphasizes organic farms and foods not for their sake alone, but for "future generations."

At heart, organic farmers are stewards of the land and managers of sustainable agriculture. This means they want the land to be viable for growing food for future generations. The small family farm, once the foundation of American society, is threatened with extinction...Organic farmers, and all promoters of sustainable agriculture, want to prevent our children from inheriting a planet in crisis...Instead, they want to create a legacy of fertile land that will produce healthy food for future generations.[16]

Organic supporters may have started out as radicals or environmentalists, but they graduated into middle-class, educated shoppers who consider quality when purchasing food. Similarly, organic suppliers may have started out as small entrepreneur-led businesses, but they have grown into medium-size corporations...It is this combination of consumer demand and corporate involvement that is making organics accessible to the mainstream in the twenty-first century.[17]

Some people may be skeptical about how organic methods can feed the same number of people as conventional methods. For millennia, however, communities have subsisted on their own private small farms, which would have been organic up until the latter half of the previous century. In many areas of the world, small organic farming is still the norm, and is even being taught by some groups of Westerners for the provision of both food and wages in some impoverished areas.

The availability of organic food is becoming more prevalent as the results of conventional agriculture have started to be realized. While conventional foods are only getting worse, organic alternatives are continually appearing on the natural foods market and only increasing its potential. Small, local growers are filling niche markets for natural food when they would have had difficulty competing with conventional mass-producers had they used conventional agriculture methods. That the nationwide demand for organic food is said to be growing by a tremendous thirty percent yearly is heartening news.

Let us again refer to an expert to hear his opinion on the organic movement. Evidently, the forecast is for its "permanent growth" since it is fulfilling its design—which is to produce specialized quantities of high-quality food.

Organic is no longer a niche market, and its popularity is not just a fad. It represents a steady, permanent growth driven by the demand of shoppers demonstrating their willingness to pay for the benefits of flavor, quality, health, nutrition, and food.[18]

Organic farming was never designed to produce large volumes of food at low prices. It was designed to produce high-quality, nutritious food while respecting the health of people and animals.[19]

Countless whole-food stores, natural markets, and organic delicatessens and restaurants are opening up around the United States, especially in particular areas of the country. Many grocery stores and wholesalers are regularly carrying organic and natural products, and some standard stores have dedicated entire sections of aisles to alternative products. The blossoming availability and selection of fresh and natural foods is very encouraging. As long as a physical and philosophical link to the countryside remains, one benefit of largely-populated regions is the opportunity for a wide variety of locally grown and locally prepared foods and other natural supplies. Many United States cities have started *Edible Communities*® publications which showcase local food growers and retailers; the material in my own region's magazine is impressive.[20] Gratefully, enough entrepreneurs and consumers in the last few decades have been diligent in sticking to their standards when organic food and household products were the minority, so that now shopping, living, and eating naturally are made easier for the rest of us.

Chapter Seventeen

Definitions for Agriculture

"Organic food isn't a luxury. It's how food is supposed to be."[1]
—Shane Heaton

BEFORE FURTHER EXPLANATION about which foods are better and worse for purchase and consumption, here are a few definitions to give you an idea of what options are available.

Conventional agriculture: From a quick internet search to see how conventional agriculture has been labeled, the following phrases were used: "characterized by mechanization;" "emphasis on maximizing productivity and profitability;"[2] "intensive mass animal farming;" synthetic fertilizers, pesticides, and applicants; genetic engineering; prevalent for the last sixty years since World War II; and, the method characteristic of the twentieth century.

Dr. Jordan Rubin tells about what has changed in agriculture since World War II and what the consequences are to our soil. Sterility is serious business because it will not allow for the creation of more life.

We sterilize our agricultural soil with pesticides and herbicides, destroying beneficial and harmful bacteria alike, even harming plants' natural immune systems. Our food used to have loads of bacterial organisms which became part of the plant and which we consumed. Now, our soil is sterile; our foods are sterile; (and, in a sense, for too many, our lives are sterile)...From thousands of years up to about half-a-century ago, the American agricultural system raised fruits and vegetables in soil exceedingly rich in bacteria and other organisms. After World War II, however, these homeostatic soil organisms were displaced as a result of chemical farming and pesticide usage by big agricultural business.[3]

How do we expect our bodies to assimilate what it takes huge manufacturing facilities to process and package into "food?" God made our bodies to be remarkable, though. They are very resilient if they can even digest something that has all the nutrients taken out and countless artificial things added in. But, actually, we cannot digest those things very well; they get stuck in our intestines—hence the understanding that all disease begins in the colon. God did not create plants and animals so that they had to be altered by processing plants in industrialized nations before we could eat them. He created food that could be acquired from the garden, forest, field, and sea, and eaten directly, in that form. This is what best nourishes man. God created foods so amazingly that many good properties are lost when people try to change food, mass-produce it, or enhance it. Obviously, we bake bread and cook meat, slice fruit and chop vegetables, pour oil and sprinkle salt; we mix things, cut things, and heat things. Preparing food for ease of consumption, however, is far different, and far more necessary, than preserving food for an unnaturally long shelf life or producing food in the largest, cheapest quantities imaginable—the latter two of which are the hallmark of conventional agriculture.

In conventional agriculture, animals are given drugs and antibiotics to cover up the health problems that they acquire from feeding on a poor diet in miserable conditions. Though allopathic treatment recommends the taking of medicines as soon as problems arise, many people are wary of this practice and hesitate to follow it, preferring rather to find the root cause of any symptoms. Why, therefore, would we accept a similar allopathic-type treatment to cover up the disease symptoms in chickens and cattle, the meat of which we will afterward be ingesting?

We laugh if we hear someone say that they could live on ice cream or chocolate all of the time, yet with conventional cattle it is not much different. Feedlot cattle are fed high-fructose grains—a diet virtually foreign to their native habitat—and become very unhealthy, often developing tumors. But the conventional agriculture business doesn't change the cows' diets; instead, the cows are given antibiotics to keep them alive until the time of slaughter. This, my friends, is the kind of thinking that goes on in conventional agriculture, and it is driven primarily by the availability and profitability of the end product, never the actual integrity of the food. The conventional agriculture industry needs to be counteracted by a withdrawal of support and by the raising and/or purchasing of good quality food by informed men and women.

Conventional food producers are evidently not very proud of the processes they use. Many companies still want their food to sound homemade or natural by using words such as "nature," "Mom's," or "Grandma's" in their brand names and descriptions. The largest food companies still have emblems of classic red barns and windmills on their packaging, though their factories surely don't look that way! A picture is worth a thousand words, though, and people gravitate toward those pictures rather than reading the ingredients or researching the processes involved in making the product.

Chemical agriculture has only been "conventional," or normal, for sixty years. In the previous millennia, organic farming was conventional, or normal; it needs to become the norm again. Christians shouldn't succumb to the culture's definition of "normal" in anything; we need to work at defining *what* "normal" is.

Genetic modification: Another definition to consider is genetic modification, a process which alters the biology of foods (meats, grains, produce, and oils) at the cellular level. This is different from the widely-accepted crossing of plant or animal varieties by grafting or selective breeding. Genetic modification has relatively unknown consequences, having been permitted only since 1980, but what is known is alarming. The practice of genetic modification is not far different from the ethics of altering the cells of human biology, about which many Christians are concerned. While stem cell research deals with organisms with the capacity of living, immortal souls (unlike genetic modification), it is likewise based on inappropriate cell engineering with the potential to greatly damage human life. As Jesus said in the Gospel of Matthew, albeit specifically in mention of marriage, "What therefore God hath joined together, let not man put asunder" (Matt. 19:6).

Genetic modification violates both principles of plant reproduction given in Genesis 1:11, which reads: "And God said, Let the earth bring forth grass, the herb yielding seed, and the fruit tree yielding fruit after his kind, whose seed is in itself, upon the earth, and it was so." Joel Salatin, author of *Holy Cows and Hog Heaven*, has gleaned the following imperatives from that verse. "A. The plants should reproduce from their own seed. B. The seeds should germinate true—children should look like parents."[4] Genetically modified organisms (GMOs) are hybrid—they cannot reproduce—and are not like the parent plant—a corn plant may have genes from a fish or a tomato in it.

The ingestion of genetically modified organisms is being linked to the alteration of human organs and bodily functions and to obesity, since our digestion of GMO foods is necessarily altered by virtue of the distorted cellular biology in the plant. As stated previously, any whole entity is affected by all the parts and processes in the chain of events leading up to an end result; we cannot drastically modify the elements of God's creation (genes) and expect them to have no affect on other parts of God's creation (human biology). Many plants, especially corn and soybeans, are genetically modified for resistance to strong pesticides, so even more sprays are used than normal. Once we start to get away from God's original intent for agriculture and diet, we enter a vicious cycle that will invariably arrive at increased pollution and destruction.

An article from *Natural News* online cites a professional opinion on GMO foods; it is quoted next. The called-for moratorium will probably never be enacted as long as food giants hold the power that they do—and as long as people keep trusting and buying GMO foods.

> The American Academy of Environmental Medicine (AAEM) states, 'Genetically Modified foods have not been properly tested and pose a serious health risk. There is more than a casual association between GM foods and adverse health effects. There is causation.' The AAEM also called for a moratorium on GMO's in food and for physicians to advise their patients to avoid GM foods. Since the massive invasion of GMO's into the food supply from 1996, chronic diseases and food allergies have doubled.[5]

The crops most likely to be genetically engineered are soy, corn, canola, and cottonseed. Ingredients and oils made from these crops are extensively used in basically all processed and packaged foods, in conventional restaurant fare, and in the feed of most beef, poultry, and pork. It is believed that seventy percent of conventional processed food contains genetically-modified organisms. Since genetically engineered foods are unlikely to be disappearing from the market anytime soon, it is imperative for conscientious consumers to avoid those foods for the sake of their own health and for the sake of influencing the market away from GMOs and toward organics. Wise trends are not being supported from the top; we need to be active at the grassroots level to fight against modified food. For instance, President Obama appointed as his "food czar" the former head of company that led the way for GMO crops, and the FDA treats GMO foods as being no different from non-GMO foods.[6]

Organic agriculture: Organic food is the pure, base form that God created—raised and produced without any of the elements common to conventional agriculture. Two definitions follow, one from Annie Eicher writing for the University of California at Davis, and the other from *The Organic Food Guide*.

> [Organic agricultural practices] promote the use of renewable resources and management of biological cycles without the use of genetically modified organisms, or synthetic pesticides, herbicides, or fertilizers. Organic livestock production promotes concern for animal welfare without the use of synthetic foodstuffs, growth hormones, or antibiotics.[7]

> Organic food reduces or eliminates the typical health and safety risks associated with modern conventional (chemical) farming.[8]

Sustainable organic agriculture is "ecologically sound, economically viable, and socially just" and is "capable of maintaining productivity indefinitely."[9] As such, organic agriculture is what best stewards the earth and preserves it for the benefit of future generations. Conventional standards, on the other hand, cannot "maintain productivity indefinitely"; the earth becomes more polluted and less able to produce, and more chemical fertilizers are used as a consequence.

Transitional agriculture, a term found on some products and produce, uses organic practices but has not fulfilled the time requirements to become certified organic. Many non-certified, but organic-in-practice, companies will list their practices on their labels, such as "no growth hormones," "100% grass-fed," or "no antibiotics." These terms are not regulated by the FDA at this point and are based on trust between the producer and purchaser.

Uniform labeling for organic food was first started by the USDA in 2002. The USDA Organic Certification ensures that foods have been produced—from start to finish—with no chemical herbicides, fungicides, pesticides, or fertilizers; no sewage-based fertilizers; and no chemical or synthetic additives. The animals resulting in organic animal products have spent time grazing outdoors on organic pastures or have been fed with organic feed, and cannot have been given hormones, antibiotics, or by-products from animals. Organic produce legally cannot be genetically engineered or irradiated and has been proven to be higher in antioxidants than its conventional counterpart. Organic food is grown from completely natural sources including the soil and the feed and is manufactured naturally without chemicals. "USDA 100% Organic" means exactly what it sounds like; "USDA Organic" means that 95% of the ingredients must be of certified organic origin. "Made with organic ingredients" legally contains 70-94% certified organic ingredients. The USDA Organic certification guarantees only the purity, not the wholesomeness of the end product, however. A food may be organic all the way from germination to packaging, and still undergo as much fractionating and processing as its conventional counterpart.

Some companies and growers will promise the same things that organic food is known for, without being certified organic, if they want to avoid the government regulations and the cost inherent with certification. These items are marketed as being completely natural and can be a good and more economical alternative to certified-organic food. "Certified Naturally Grown" is another recent and non-government-backed endorsement with essentially the same standards as USDA Organic. "Quality Assurance International" and "Oregon Tilth" are two other such endorsements of organic food. Looking for these labels can help in the search for natural products.

Organic produce has been repeatedly found to have 50-140% more individual nutrients (calcium, magnesium, Vitamin A, Vitamin C, etc.) than their non-organic counterparts. Organic food isn't somehow extraordinary—the nutrients in conventional food are continually and drastically dropping, leaving organic foods the way God made them. In one study period of forty-seven years, the USDA found that the calcium in conventional broccoli had dropped by fifty percent, the potassium in collard greens had dropped by fifty-eight percent, and the Vitamin C in cauliflower had dropped by fifty percent.[10] Organic foods have been found to harbor fifteen percent fewer nitrates and heavy metals than their non-organic counterparts. Organic produce may cost more but it enriches health in return.

Natural ingredients: "All-natural" products usually contain nothing artificial (no additives, preservatives, flavors, or colors), but make no promise as to the origin or growing methods of the ingredients (unless it is additionally stated, as mentioned above.) Pesticides *can* be used in raising the crops used in "all-natural" products, so many labels will promise "pesticide-free" without going through certification. You should read the ingredients no matter what the front label says, and determine whether anything manmade is among them. By the way, the single word "natural" in the brand name or packaging doesn't promise anything except a vague concept. There are no regulations at this point for using the word "natural" or "all natural." Likewise, there are no regulations for the terms "traditional," "free-range," pastured," or "grass-fed"; ideally, this is as it should be, and the consumer should either be able to trust the company promising these things, or personally know enough about the product without having to read claims on packages.

Also, the words "made with" are no indicator of health value or of the purity or simplicity of ingredients. For instance, a product that promises "made with honey" can truthfully contain sugar, high fructose corn syrup, molasses, and several other sweeteners in addition to honey. Labels get away with as little information as possible. In the above scenario, there is a good reason the product does not say "100% honey-sweetened" or some such claim. The consumer must read the ingredients and pay attention to subtle words that, upon further investigation, have a misleading connotation.

Pure, natural foods are complex by virtue of God's creating them but are simple for our bodies to digest and go directly toward nourishing us. Complex foods and ingredients—by virtue of man's modification—are not at all better than natural foods. They are confusing to our bodies and hard to digest, and our bodies can only use part of what is found in any artificially processed foods. Man simply cannot improve upon God's design.

Food with anything taken out or anything added in is not natural! (By addition and subtraction, I mean stripping wheat of its bran and germ or injecting cows with hormones. Mixing together butter, eggs, honey, and wheat flour for baking a cake is not, in that sense, adding to whole foods but *combining* them.) Look at the natural world around us; God, not man, is the Creator who is blessed forever. As much as we believe that God created the world, so much should we love the natural things of His creation.

Artificial ingredients: Who would intentionally eat anything artificial—something that isn't food? Manmade ingredients just do not sound like something we should *eat*. While the foremost ingredients in a product are not artificial (wheat is not mimicked with anything manmade, for instance), there can be so many artificial additives and processes applied that the whole nature of the original food is changed. Much conventionally produced food today contains artificial colors, artificial flavors, artificial sweeteners, artificially altered oils, and synthetic hormones and chemicals. Artificial chemical compounds are not metabolized by our bodies because they are not recognized as something our body can assimilate. Artificial is defined as humanly contrived, misleading, and unnatural. The word artifice, from which artificial is derived, has an even worse connotation, meaning insincerity, trickery, or pretense.

For artificial flavors, chemists synthetically duplicate the molecular structure of the molecules that give flavor to real foods. If we eat almonds—the example used below—we obtain benzaldehyde as an element of a whole food. If we eat food with synthetic benzaldehyde, we are not getting it as part of a whole food and we get the harmful effects of the chemical combination. Benzaldehyde used in fragrances is thought to be damaging to the liver and kidneys—and flavorings are no different. It is explained here how artificial flavors are developed:

> To make an artificial flavor, a flavor chemist (called a flavorist) in a laboratory has to select and blend the right chemical compounds in the right amounts to simulate the natural flavor. And to obtain and concentrate the natural flavoring compounds, someone in another laboratory or factory has to extract or distill them from the raw plant or animal materials...

> For example, the primary natural flavor compound in almonds is benzaldehyde; when our taste receptors come across a molecule of benzaldehyde, they shout "almond" to our brains. So some food manufacturers use synthesized (laboratory-made) benzaldehyde as an artificial almond flavoring.[11]

Modern food is adulterated, poisoned, and corrupted but is described as fortified, enriched, or improved.[12] Manufacturers can claim anything on their packaging and can put a nice label on any type of food, no matter how inferior it is. For instance, many products sport the claim of "sugar-free" as if to sound healthier, when in reality, the artificial sweeteners used are far worse even than refined cane sugar. We need to find out the truth about how things are made and understand that deception—such as pictures of happy children eating very harmful food—is strategic in getting consumers to buy junk.

Imitation and deception are wrong—and are what Satan does to imitate God and get people to like sinful things. It is a Christian principle that our lives should be pure, candid, and genuine—without deceit. While I would not go so far as claiming that imitation of food is blatant sin, I think the above principles apply. Imitation is deceptive and cannot be as good as the real thing. Honesty and sincerity are the marks of an upright person and are the marks of true advertising of wholesome food.

I am thankful that a foundation of truth exists in advertising, such that products are mandated to say whether they are artificially flavored. The ingredient list is the most truthful part of the packaging, though artificial ingredients may legally be hidden behind such obscure listings as "natural flavors."

Thankfully, alternative products exist which are produced by companies who care more about the integrity of food than the volume and bottom line of their corporation. At least the ingredients within a food product or food company are generally consistent, making it easier on the buyer. Manufacturers that will use artificial flavors and colors usually use hydrogenated oils, MSG, enriched flour, and preservatives. Manufacturers that understand a problem with any one of these ingredients will strive to keep the remainder of their ingredients pure and natural as well.

However, any level of truth in advertising only tells us the ingredients of the end product, not the whole manufacturing process or what the food does to us. Truth would be saying that the artificial flavor in such-and-such food is known to cause hyperactivity, or that the sugars will decay your teeth, or that chemicals and additives are addictive.[13] Truth in advertising might be exemplified as happy people eating fresh strawberries, but it is not happy people eating strawberry toaster-tarts. Why? Because refined flours, refined sugars, refined oils, and artificial flavors and colors have been documented to lead to nervous, emotional, and digestive disorders, *not* a sense of well-being that only natural food gives.

God's foods need no advertising; they grow colorfully on bushes and trees or graze peacefully in meadows and mountains. Manmade foods, though, have to compete with each other by patents, by the pictures on their boxes, and by the supposed claims of having more fiber or more vitamin C than the next box.

Poison: Dictionaries define poison as a substance that causes injury, illness, or death; to have a harmful influence on; to corrupt. Many ingredients that are used in food manufacturing are harmful in large quantities or with prolonged use and could veritably be called poisonous. Pure, healthy foods are only beneficial in larger quantities, but not so with processed foods.

Have you ever seen the movie "Arsenic and Old Lace," where friends and family members were trying to poison each other with laced wine? Though not a favorite of mine, this film can provide an illustration. To the unsuspecting, the wine looked appealing and would have tasted as it customarily did. To the knowledgeable, it was known to be harmful and mingled with the substance of ominous purposes. Motives and potency aside, much food in the grocery store is similar. To the naïve, harmful food seems harmless, even pleasing. Informed minds, on the contrary, will look at the same food and distinguish pollution and toxicity mingled throughout it.

Dr. Colbert says that toxins in food are mostly found in caffeine, the fat in conventionally-grown animal products, trans-fats, food additives, drugs, and medicines. "Much of our air is contaminated. Most of our water is tainted. Our food usually contains toxins."[14] Fresh fruits and vegetables, conventionally grown, are also contaminated with toxins in the form of residual pesticides. The pesticides that are the greatest threat to human health are the same ones that are most-used, according to the Environmental Protection Agency.[15]

As conscientious consumers, we need to avoid a litany of products if we want to avoid conventional, artificial, and poisonous substances. There is much hope, however, in the accessibility of alternative, natural, organic, pure, and wholesome foods. Mercifully, we have a choice not to eat toxic food. We do, however, need to keep thinking, keep buying responsibly, and keep voting responsibly, in order to retain the freedom to eat well. The United States government (mainly the FDA) is certainly not protecting American citizens, but is allowing and promoting the use of poisons, from fertilizers to food additives to drugs. We need to do our own research and be faithful about applying our findings to our purchasing decisions.

Nourishment: Nourishing food supplies what is necessary for promoting and sustaining growth, supporting and maintaining life, and fostering health. Nourishing food needs to be eaten in its pure form lest its qualities be compromised. Additives in food take away the nourishing benefits of the original foods rather than being neutral additions.

If we eat part of what is nourishing and part of what is poisonous (poisonous in large quantities or in accumulation), that is schizophrenic. Ingesting part nourishment and part artifice is like reading the Bible and agnostic literature in equal part and hoping to end up with a Holy-Spirit-sanctified mind; it will hardly happen. If we want to be healthy, we need to eat healthy foods, which means animals and plants that have been eating or taking in healthy things—cows and chickens eating green grass instead of animal parts, plants taking in pure air and mineral-rich soil instead of chemicals, and biblically-clean creatures taking in the same kinds of food that God intended for mankind to eat.

Diet: Our regular consumption of food and drink; our habitual nourishment; our established pattern of eating. Diet is also defined as a specific regimen or prescribed eating plan, or the act of restricting intake.

A "diet" should not be an extreme deprivation plan that you use for a little while and then return to normal, poor eating habits. A regulated time on a cleansing diet can be profitable, but our ongoing eating patterns should be carefully established and regulated. One's diet, or "habitual nourishment," should not be made light of. If a diet is followed by default, it needs some attention. If our diet is followed by intention, it needs to be met with deference.

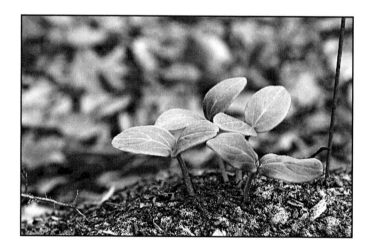

Chapter Eighteen

Categories of American Diet

"Americans have more food to eat than any other people,
and more diets to keep them from eating it."[1]

—Anonymous

DRIVING THROUGH A fast-food restaurant, a man quickly exchanges a few dollars for a thin deep-fried hamburger topped with a soft white bun, sugary condiments, and vegetables that consist of pickles, ketchup, and deep-fried potatoes. Sitting down to their old oak table, a family asks divine blessing over a meal consisting of that season's wild venison steaks rubbed with herbs, a salad showcasing produce from the farmers' market, and hearty homemade bread with butter. Traveling abroad, a couple dresses up for dinner at a renowned gourmet restaurant that promises to have every ethnic delicacy sautéed to perfection, every flavor meticulously blended with the next, and every garnish artistically displayed. Hovering over a kettle in her humble kitchen, a woman on a foreign continent stirs the same kinds of broth, grains, root crops, and legumes that her ancestors have been growing and eating for centuries, and then ladles out the soup to her waiting guests. These are some of the wonders of the world.

God created a diversity of food in every climate—all nutritious and particularly suited to the people dwelling in each climate. People have used certain nutritious combinations together for centuries: fish, taro, and tropical fruit; wild game, corn, and berries; beef and wheat; lamb, potatoes, and garden vegetables; beans and rice. World cultures typically cook with standard, traditional blends of proteins and starches. God has designed balanced combinations of nutrients to flourish in the same climate; and native peoples have utilized and thrived on these combinations.

Many ancient cultures have believed—have known—that the right foods act as medicine. If foods change us, we must choose the right foods. If we use the right foods, our ailments can be alleviated. The Greek Hippocrates, father of Western medicine and to whom the statement "food is your best medicine" is attributed, elaborated on that thought as follows. While medical practitioners still use a form of the Hippocratic Oath, this short expression would be a wise model for food manufacturers and home kitchens.

> Each of the substances of a man's diet acts upon his body and changes it in some way, and upon these changes his whole life depends.[2]

America, the breadbasket of the world, grows most foods on her own land. Specialty preparations that are still done in other countries are imported. With this variety at our fingertips, we have no excuse for making the best possible use of the nutrients available. Superfluity of choices, however, can be overwhelming, and Americans frequently choose what is the most marketed and most popular. We have taken the combinations we are used to, such as beef and wheat, and refined them as much as possible. There is a standard American diet, but all Americans do not, and do not need to, eat that way. We are blessed with more variety and choice than many other places in the world, and there are many various types of diets from which we can readily choose.

Following are a few attributes of some of the most common diets or particular ways of eating. While my commentary is unavoidably influenced by my own decisions and experience, I hope this chapter will give a helpful background for readers who are trying for the first time to change their habits. As always, good principles need to be applied: evaluate information, make a thoughtful decision, and be disciplined to follow the dictates of that decision while being willing to learn more.

Standard American Diet: As Dr. Jordan Rubin explains in *Patient, Heal Thyself,* departure from tradition seems to be the prevailing American standard. His claim of fifty-five percent newfangled food seems completely plausible after a glance at an average American supermarket or restaurant.

> Before the advent of widespread modern agriculture, the human diet consisted mostly of fruits, vegetables, wild grains and seeds, fish, and meat from wild animals. No matter how far we have progressed socially and technologically, our bodies still crave the foods of our ancestors...We have departed so far from the wisdom of our forefathers that fully 55 percent of the American diet is "new food" not eaten by our ancestors.[3]

With the lack of large metropolitan areas in the Rocky Mountain region where we live, and the local emphasis on fitness and outdoor recreation, it is easy for me to forget that most Americans *do* consume and overeat the unhealthful foods that fill supermarkets and restaurants. The statistics for amounts of junk food sold and statistics for climbing disease rates are both alarming—and are very real. Though I have always lived in a quite health-conscious area of the nation and have had the luxury to be acquainted with many health-conscious friends, I have only to pick up magazine advertisements or take a trip to be reminded that the Standard American Diet still very much prevails.

Something must be contributing to the tragic rise in disease that has taken precedence since the early twentieth century. While people used to die from war, malnutrition, or agedness, people now die from an unbalanced diet—this occurring in America, the "breadbasket of the world" and the nation with the largest healthcare system. The newfangled characteristics of now-standard American eating habits are the following: processed food products, excess sugar, refined grain, hydrogenated oil, synthetic additives, and exceedingly low fruit and vegetable intake. Cooked, processed foods lack the enzymes necessary to supply our bodies with life-giving energy to maintain our organs and digestive system. Processed foods are notoriously high in refined sugars, refined sodium, and refined oils—the very culprits linked to many diseases, and the very ingredients (sugar, salt and fat) which occur rarely in the realm of nature. While national associations such as the American Heart Association and American Cancer Society advocate the limiting of animal fats (in dairy products and red meat), these omissions are not the answer.

While it is tempting to do so, we cannot think of the standard American diet as "normal." The standard American diet is foreign to history and to most of the world, not to mention foreign to our bodies. Traditional societies have eaten similar proportions of dairy products and red meat as Americans do today; *however*, traditional peoples did not have the diseases that today are associated with red meat and the fat in dairy products. Meat and milk from animals raised naturally on grass is much healthier for human consumption and never used to lead to heart disease and cancer as people claim it does now. To the credit of national research, today's conventionally raised meat and milk *do* seem to lead to heart disease and cancer—but they do not have to, if we would only eat organic, grass-fed animal products.

The solution for promoting health is not to eliminate what has always, historically, been consumed, but to look at what else has changed: the methods of raising and processing meat, milk, and eggs, coupled with the other poor aspects of our diet. Instead of suggesting the use of skim milk and margarine in brownies, nutritionists should suggest that no refined flour or sugar be used—for those are equally detrimental to our bodies. In fact, organic butter and whole milk are some of the most healthful products in existence and should be used frequently. Instead of frying up "lean," conventional chicken breasts in soybean oil, it should be suggested that organic chicken is cooked in olive or coconut oil. Instead of hormones and heart disease, your body will then be given good protein and boosted immunity.

The American diet is too *white*—an instance where pure white is awful, and neither good nor beneficial. The coconut in one pudding box I looked at had been bleached and then artificial color was added back in to the pudding mix. Conventional brands of feminine napkins are bleached with dioxins, which are highly toxic and carcinogenic. The list could go on. The predilection for having things white has gotten out of control.

Usually our Christian connotation of white is "pure," but not so in food. When God cleanses our hearts and forgives our sin, the Bible says we are whiter than snow, but when man tries to make food better by whitening it, he ruins what God created. The nutrients in food, especially vitamins, are where the color lies, and vice versa. We need to restore the practice of loving what God created and using it in the state He created it. Christians need to be disciplined in not succumbing to the peer pressure of everyone around them who eats the standard diet and makes light of those who think about their food. By far, the easiest place to succumb to the American diet is the eating of empty, dead calories found in white sugar and white flour.

The standard American diet is relatively easy to find. It consists of practically everything that is easily acquired in the center aisles of most grocery stores and restaurants that is neither 1) a simple food like bananas or walnuts or green salad, nor 2) advertised as an alternative product. Alternative products are foods that have been manufactured in avoidance of the typical culprits in conventional agriculture. They will be advertised as organic, no trans-fats, no hormones, no hydrogenated oils, fresh, local, raw, sustainable, grass-fed, or many other descriptors of healthy food. The standard American diet consists of starchy, processed carbohydrates, fatty meats, artificial additives, harmful oils, too few vegetables, and too little fiber. We are talking about a difference between the popular foods of technology and the timeless foods of our ancestors. The standard American diet has become the norm in the United States and one has to think and look carefully in order to avoid it and replace it with traditional, nourishing foods.

Raw Foods: Many of the people most interested in a healthy lifestyle will consume only raw, vegetarian foods—fruits, vegetables, nuts, seeds, sprouted grains and legumes, and vegetable oils. This is understood as the diet whereby the life-giving matter of fruits and vegetables, nuts and legumes, are most able to directly nourish and powerfully cleanse the body. Many people in America today credit their thriving health to a raw or primarily-raw vegetarian diet.

While raw, living foods are profusely nutritious, and would be helpful for a period of cleansing from disease or for weight loss, a completely raw diet is neither a historical nor biblical pattern. Subsistence farmers and hunter-gatherer tribes in temperate climates could hardly expect to have fresh produce year-round. Many cultures with a marked degree of health, worldwide, consist primarily on provisions from animals. Without eating a solely raw diet, foods in their raw form are to be desired above heated foods, when possible; for example, raw milk and raw honey are better than that pasteurized.

Though He at first gave Adam "every herb-bearing seed" for food, after mankind's Fall, God soon established the consumption of animal products with instructions about cooking and preparing them (Ex. 12:8–9). As the Old Testament repeatedly gives examples, flour and breads were made from grain, and animal flesh was roasted. Raw foods, then, were not at all the ultimate diet of ancient times. Though the Israelites lived in the "land flowing with milk and honey," a region capable of supplying many fresh fruits and vegetables, God made it clear that Israelites were to cook and eat bread and meat (such as at the Passover and other feasts.)

For the Israelites, God prescribed certain animals for consumption and forbad others. We should notice that animals were classified as clean and unclean at the time of their entering Noah's ark, which was during the time when man ate only the herb-bearing seed, and which was prior to God's allowing animals for man's food. God retained the same clean-and-unclean criteria in His laws for the Israelites as He had earlier expressed to Noah and his plant-eating family.

Vegetarian: Many people will consume primarily plant foods for reasons either of health or conscience. "Vegetarian" can mean a whole range of things, from avoiding meat, or avoiding meat and eggs, or avoiding meat, milk, and eggs. "Vegan" means consuming no animal products whatsoever, and often includes a practice of having a household free of products that have come from animals. The description "vegetarian," however, denotes nothing about how natural or unrefined the products are.

Biblical evidence against a vegetarian diet is similar to that mentioned above regarding raw foods. Jesus ate bread and fish and fed it to thousands gathered to hear Him expound the testimony of God. The Apostle Paul uses milk and meat as analogies of spiritual strength; the list could go on. Animal products are not at all foreign to Scripture. Even broader than the testimony from Bible times is evidence from across the globe. Peoples with mostly vegetarian diets are weaker and less productive than those who have eaten wholesome meat and dairy products.

The general proportion of nutrients from healthful peoples around the world has consisted of (calories coming from) 40% protein, 40% fats, and 20% carbohydrates. This is quite difficult to accomplish with any combination of raw, vegan, or vegetarian foods.

The Standard American Diet consists of (calories coming from) 40% carbohydrates, 40% fats, and 20% protein; this statistic is moving in the direction of a less-meat-intensive diet and has shown only detrimental results.

The book *Nourishing Traditions* indicates that animal fats are the only source of A and D vitamins and that animal protein is the only complete protein in the world. Animal products are important for keeping the body's acid-alkaline balance.[4]

Dr. Jordan Rubin gives expert insight on historical diets in his books. Discussing the vegetarian diet, he explains that an emphasis on fruits and vegetables for a short period can decrease the body's "toxic burden" and cleanse the body. The vital nutrients lacking when animal foods are completely deprived from the diet, however, are necessary for longevity and without these elements there may be "deadly consequences." Meat-eating tribes are found to be longer-lived than vegetarian societies, the doctor says, as proven by anthropological study.[5]

Mediterranean: The Mediterranean diet is the cuisine of the countries surrounding the Mediterranean Sea, and is becoming popular in certain coastal areas of the United States, especially California. This diet is frequently mentioned with regard to its health benefits, since people from these countries have low rates of heart disease. Though the Southern Europeans, Middle Easterners, and Northern Africans in lands bordering the Sea consume a high percentage of oil, this oil is in a pure, cold-pressed form and is loaded with heart-healthy omega-3 fatty acids. The fat in their diet comes primarily from the monounsaturated and polyunsaturated fats of olives and olive oil, nuts and seeds, and fish. In addition to good oils and the fat from fish—one of the most nutritious animal foods—the Mediterranean climate boasts an abundant availability of fresh fruits and vegetables and legumes which are incorporated as a mainstay of nearly every meal.

The unique aspect of the Mediterranean diet (a.k.a. French diet or Sonoma diet) is eating foods in combination. Low-glycemic-index foods and high-glycemic-index foods (based on how they raise blood sugar) are eaten together. Mediterranean meals consist of either mostly protein or mostly carbohydrates, not together. Americans, on the contrary, usually eat high-glycemic carbohydrate foods alone, such as pizza with chips and soda, without balancing them out with low-glycemic foods to lessen the effect of the former on blood sugar. Americans often eat carbohydrates with large portions of protein, such as hamburgers with buns and fries or steak with potatoes.

Author Michel Montignac advises a wiser approach to eating high-glycemic carbohydrates. (His excellent and popular book *The French Diet* gives menu plans to aid in the practice of this proposal.)

...You can eat carbohydrates with a high GI [glycemic index] but only when you balance them out. This means that during the course of your meal, a food with a high GI has to be balanced by a food with a low GI and a high fiber content.[6]

The Mediterranean diet is worthy of consideration and can be a most pleasurable way to "diet" for weight loss and health gain, as it is relatively flexible but loaded with good nutrition. As long as the right foods are eaten, quantity is hardly an issue, because good fats and oils and fresh fruits and vegetables never contribute to excess body fat. In your shopping, looking for foods associated with the Mediterranean countries can be a good indicator of healthfulness of food.

Kosher: Certified kosher foods uphold the Jewish rabbinical standards, codifying the laws that God gave to the Israelites. Specifically, kosher laws regulate what parts and kinds of meat can be used and how they are prepared. Kosher foods will have no animal products from biblically unclean animals—such as gelatin from pig's feet, or pork fat in beef preparations. While kosher foods do not stray from the commandments from God to the Israelites, these foods are not necessarily healthy or wholesome, since they can still be very refined.

Low-carbohydrate, low-fat, or calorie-counting diets: These trends are good in the sense that they realize the excess of, and consequence of, refined starches and oils and fatty meats in our standard cuisine. Going without starches for a time can be helpful for weight loss. Many people eat an imbalanced proportion of starchy carbohydrates to other fruits and vegetables, fats and proteins, and a healthier balance could be achieved. Wholesome kinds of grains and oils, however, are very nutritious and necessary for us and do contribute to good health and proper weight levels. Eliminating a major and necessary part of the diet is not good long-term. Plus, calorie-counting diets make food seem like our "enemy."[7] People often bounce back to poor eating habits after strict dieting periods. We should, rather, restrict intake of unhealthy foods and have a balanced diet of the most nutritious foods all of the time. It is best to stick as closely as possible to a traditional (pre-1900) diet, which was lower in carbohydrates and higher in proteins and good fats than the weight-promoting Standard American Diet.

In *The French Diet*, Mr. Montignac says that Americans have "decreased their caloric intake by as much as 30%," but that two-thirds of this country's population is overweight. Half of the overweight population is said to be obese—which is a higher proportion than that in any other country.[8] The same author goes on to describe some important, little-known facts about calories:

...The energy factor of a food—its caloric content—is not the deciding factor in weight gain, as has long been believed. It is the nutritional content that is important, because it determines the type of metabolic reaction a food causes.[9]

Biblical: The diet of the Hebrew people was obviously kosher, as well as being influenced by the indigenous foods of the Mediterranean region. The Bible records, to name a few things, figs, grapes, palm and apple trees, almonds, fish, wheat, barley, butter, and honey. Nutrient-dense plant and animal foods used alongside a diet of whole grains and clean meats would have been akin to the most healthful foods that nutritionists recommend today. Many things eaten by the Israelites are today regarded as super-foods, such as pomegranates, olives and olive oil, flaxseed, and goat's milk. Some of the spices and seasonings commonly used in Bible times have some of the most potent antioxidants known today, such as cumin, cinnamon, hyssop, and honey. While countries surrounding the nation of Israel all had somewhat similar Mediterranean-type diets, God gave His people certain dietary and cleanliness laws that, when followed, protected them from the "diseases of the Egyptians" (Ex. 15:26; Deut. 7:15). These were promises made specifically to the Hebrews in that era, but they can at least inform and instruct us about health in God's economy.

In the New Covenant, as it was stated in chapter four, there is no *specific* set of dietary rules prescribed for the lawful obedience of God's people. No such expectation should be inferred from mine or any other treatment of a God-honoring diet. The historical narratives in Scripture do not serve as a foundation of doctrine—such as implying that we must eat hyssop and figs and barley—but the narratives do serve as an example of what God approved or censured and when God blessed or withheld blessing. Many of the food-related patterns and principles in the Bible are helpful to understand. There are doctrines that govern our appetites, however. Taken together, the beliefs that God created the natural environment, that the earth is for man's dominion, that our bodies are Christ's temples, and that our lives are for glorifying God should necessarily give shape to a paradigm for food and eating.

It is written that all of Scripture is instructive for a faithful and holy Christian life. One principle of proper biblical interpretation is that the reader understands the historical setting into which God inspired the authors to speak or write His message to the people. So, when we read what God says in the Bible about the provision of food, the blessing of sustenance, and the harvest of crops, we should understand the time, place, and the natural and social environment about which He revealed His wisdom. The ancient Hebrew and Greco-Roman cultures were the context into which Jesus Christ came and the setting from which He deigned to teach His disciples, multiply the loaves and fishes, dine with the publicans, and tell parables about grain, vineyards, fig trees, and mustard seeds.

Traditional: What is eaten today is no longer traditional. So many things have changed, that food is hardly what food used to be. Food nourished our ancestors, but it's killing us today. What we eat now is hardly food, some would argue. What our ancestors ate is what we should be eating, many contend. The only way to regain the good health that our forefathers and foremothers often enjoyed is not to step back in time, but to step into their barns and pantries, fields and kitchens.

The harsh truth proclaimed by Dr. Jordan Rubin in this quotation should make Americans ashamed of themselves. While there are many dangerous foods that we should not be eating, there remains much hope and much potential. We can, by God's grace, still choose the "foods of our Creator", the "diets that our ancestors ate," and the foods that "nourished the world's healthiest peoples."

> Most Americans simply do not eat the nutritious diets that our own ancestors ate to remain healthy and live long, disease-free lives. Instead, we have strayed from the foods of our Creator, foods that at one time nourished the world's healthiest peoples. We have altered the Maker's intent, and we have allowed food to become our idol. We are becoming fat, sick, and sedentary. I know it's harsh. I also know it's true, and what all of us need to know is a lot more truth and a lot less fluff. The kind of things that pass for food today—what we choose for table fare—are pathetic![10]

Diets of the world before the twentieth century have largely consisted of unprocessed, unadulterated natural foods: meat that was grass-fed, not feedlot-raised; whole grains often soaked, sometimes ground, but never refined-then-"enriched;" pure fats and oils—never hydrogenated or pasteurized; animals from the wilderness and sea; fruits and nuts from orchards; and vegetables and seeds from fields.

God designed the geography and ecology of His universe so that complete nutrient combinations are found in every region. Today, we eat whatever we like, transported from anywhere in the world. While the wide selection can be a benefit, it is often a detriment since we only choose what we like—usually in the forms of refined grains and sugars—rather than what would nourish us.

It really does seem ridiculous to strip food of nutrients then wonder why we get sick, as this author of a natural-food cookbook notes:

> Someday we, if we live that long, will look back in wonder at the 'old dark days of unenlightenment' when food was systematically stripped of the very elements which gave it nutrient value.[11]

Actually, manufacturers get away with stripping and refining food because they reduce its elements to grams of protein, grams of sugar, daily percentage of vitamin C, and number of calories. "Nutrition Facts" may sound wise and good to the average consumer, but if the food product is not made with whole foods, its nutrient elements are in reality very scarce in comparison. The standards that the Nutrition Fact guidelines are based on must be very flawed, for people are not staying healthy. We ought to pay more attention to traditional, nourishing, whole foods than to numbers and percentages on boxes.

Christian: Many diets are promoted; how do we know which is best? To start with, we know that foods eaten in biblical accounts are good to eat, since God's people, His Son Jesus, and Jesus' disciples ate them. We know they ate their food in a pure, wholesome form that God created and intended. People who have historically followed these guidelines have been healthiest.

For the informed person wishing to honor God with his or her choices in the most basic of human functions—eating—I submit the following. Christians must wisely evaluate the world around them—the state of health as well as the opportunities that abound. We must search out evidence from history regarding what people ate and how they thrived. We must acknowledge all biblical commands, precepts, and examples regarding diet. Then, we must combine our data in a humble, understanding way as we seek a lifestyle that will promote, into the future, multi-generational health, productivity, and dominion. We must seek a poison-free diet in order to be the best stewards of our bodies, God's instruments for dominion—and the best stewards of the earth, God's arena for dominion.

Christians should "understand the times." To do this, we must be concerned with the past, the present, and the future. In the area of health and nutrition, concern is applied by learning from the past, navigating the present, and planning for the future in every dietary choice we make.

All research, studies, and tests across the world and throughout history point to one two-fold truth: we should eat what God created and in its purest form. God created plants and animals "very good," but man's rebellious nature permeates his actions and, often unknowingly, attacks the purity and wellness of creation. The Christian's quest is to eliminate the remnants of sinfulness in our practices and choices and to restore everything in our lives via Christ's redemption of His creation. Whatever "diet" is chosen, this remains: let it be pure, wholesome, and simple. Such a rule will be the best start on the road to a nutritious, natural lifestyle.

Chapter Nineteen

Macro-and Micronutrients

"While nature is nurturing; additives are addictive. Wholesome food makes wholesome bodies; chemical-laden food makes chemical-laden bodies."[1]

—Renée DeGroot

MACRONUTRIENTS ARE THE elements that we need in large quantities for survival. The macronutrients of carbohydrates, protein, and fat supply our quota of calories and, in turn, supply energy for our bodies to function. Micronutrients, as their name implies, are nutrients necessary in small quantities and are better known as vitamins and minerals. Micronutrients help produce enzymes and hormones and supply vitality for our bodies.

There are good sources of carbohydrates, protein, and fat, as well as less-than-desirable sources. Is this not the way that the whole of God's world operates? There are things that promote well-doing and things that promote wrong-doing; there are "instruments of righteousness" and "instruments of unrighteousness," and we are told to make the right choices (Rom. 6:13, 19 and Gal. 6:7).

There are estimated to be forty-five essential nutrients that the body requires and that come from sources outside the body (i.e. food). When we eat a narrow range of food—and the typical narrow range usually consists of food all but depleted of its nutrient value—we are asking for trouble and usually end up with trouble. Following are just a few preliminary guidelines, in the form of a list, about understanding and choosing foods; first, the macronutrients are discussed and then individual food groups, such as spices and teas, which contain micronutrients.

He sendeth the springs into the valleys, which run among the hills. They give drink to every beast of the field: the wild asses quench their thirst. By them shall the fowls of the heaven have their habitation, which sing among the branches. He watereth the hills from his chambers: the earth is satisfied with the fruit of thy works. He causeth the grass to grow for the cattle, and herb for the service of man: that he may bring forth food out of the earth; And wine that maketh glad the heart of man, and oil to make his face to shine, and bread which strengtheneth man's heart.

—Psalm 104:10–15

Carbohydrates: Carbohydrates are found in grains, other starches, and, to a lesser extent, fruits and vegetables. Carbohydrates provide fuel, energy, and power for the body. Grains and starches are wholesome and instrumental to a proper diet; however, caution is needed. Bread and flour products are produced today in an unnatural and divergent way from the centuries-old way of eating them. Whereas flour used to be ground whole or cooked whole and often soaked beforehand, today this has almost completely changed. Refined, enriched flour greatly heightens blood sugar, and for this reason, products made with it are quite addictive; not only that, but they are difficult for the body to digest and supply few useful nutrients. Refining and enriching, while the terms may sound profitable, are a ruinous process of stripping most of the fiber and vitamin content from grain kernels, then adding back in a small and practically useless amount of vitamins and minerals. Americans get twenty percent more of their calories from carbohydrates than they need to—and most of this from refined flour products. Consequently, carbohydrates are the most overdone food group in our diets. Processed, starchy, or sugary foods, while supplying energy, supply it temporarily without giving lasting rejuvenation and nourishment to the body. Have you noticed that while you might eat beef jerky, apple slices, a glass of milk, or carrot sticks until you are satisfied, it is too easy to munch continually on crackers, cookies, potato chips, pretzels, or popcorn? Processed foods spike blood sugar quickly, causing a sudden drop afterward and leaving you feeling like you need more of the same snack. Whole grains and minimally-processed whole grain products are much less addictive and much healthier at the same time.

Carbohydrate foods can be measured by how much they influence blood sugar. The amount that blood sugar, or glycemia, is raised by a certain food is indicated by the glycemic index (GI). This index was briefly mentioned in my description of the Mediterranean diet. The list of carbohydrates with a high GI is comprised of sugars, processed grains, root vegetables, and variations of these (such as corn syrup, honey, jam, sweetened canned fruit, pretzels, bagels, breads, cold cereal, crackers, pasta, rice, French fries, chips, and potatoes). Most whole or dried fruits, vegetables, cooked whole grains, nuts, and legumes have a low to very low GI. The glycemic scale has a range of ten to one hundred and ten points. Something of beneficial note—since it greatly supports the principles discussed so far—is that the more food is processed or changed, the higher the GI climbs. For instance, solid dark chocolate (such as 85% cocoa) comes in forty-five points lower than a highly-sweetened milk chocolate bar. This difference is significant—nearly half of the range on the GI. Maple syrup, while still considered high, registers forty-five points lower than corn syrup. Brown rice and white rice have a difference of forty points, and wild rice fifteen points lower than brown rice. Whole wheat pasta and white flour pasta have a difference of thirty points.[2]

The French Diet by Mr. Montignac explains carbohydrates and the glycemic index in great detail. It is really very obvious where overeating and extra weight comes from—imbalanced blood sugar that fools the body into thinking it needs more of the same refined carbohydrates.

> We have seen all too clearly where an emphasis on carbohydrates leads, especially the refined variety: a spike in blood sugar levels that stimulates hunger and encourages overeating and obesity.[3]

Note that processed grain products act just like sugars in the bloodstream—in their raising of blood sugar as well as their damage to the body. Wholesome carbohydrates contain nutrients that slow down the effect on blood sugar, nourish the body rather than providing empty calories, and generally provide balance instead of spikes in the diet.

Protein: Protein fuels the building and repair of muscles and bodily organs and is primarily found in meat, poultry, fish, cheese, eggs, legumes, and sprouted vegetables. It is very important to receive any animal protein from organic sources. The whole nature of meat or eggs is changed when grown conventionally. The fats become unhealthy for us, and the hormones and nitrates mess with our bodies. When grazed on pastures, however, grass-fed animals are healthy and produce healthy meat, milk, and eggs. Many nutritionists believe that animal products are the most important thing to buy organic or natural, much more so than organic grains, vegetables, or fruits. Conventional grains and produce are genetically modified and sprayed with pesticides, but conventionally-grown meats, eggs, and milk are modified even more harmfully and fundamentally by unnatural farming procedures and the animals' battles against filth and disease. Americans need more of good, clean proteins in their diets. Organ meats are high in minerals and many people swear by their nutrition, while others doubt their worth (hearkening back to God's commands to the Israelites). It is known, though, that pollutants gather in animal organs; if eaten, it is wise to buy organic versions.

In *The 150 Healthiest Foods on Earth*, the author gives the following assertion. Cheese, which can be an excellent protein, can be extremely unhealthful depending on how it was made:

> The whole thing with cheese is this: It's all about the source. Unfortunately, the generic name 'cheese' covers an awful lot of territory. Just as 'carbs' include lollipops and cauliflower, the 'cheese' section of the deli is a pretty big umbrella, containing everything from phenomenally wonderful natural cheeses made from the raw and unpasteurized milk of sheep and goats to single-sliced 'cheese foods' that bear absolutely no resemblance to anything that should ever be put into the human body.[4]

The source and the steps involved in food's production make all the difference in the world, as evidenced by the quotations above and below. A single word like 'cheese' or 'steak' is hardly a valid descriptor of food anymore, just as the words 'music' or 'love' have been lately used to encompass an ever-widening range of worldly notions. Until good and viable words are reclaimed to mean what they used to mean, we will need to know more than one vague word about our food. 'Beef' is not nearly enough information for a conscientious buyer. Where was it raised; what did it eat?

More wisdom from Michael Pollan, quoted from *In Defense of Food*, applies to the subject at hand. I appreciate his reservation that if a steer has not eaten whole and traditional food, its meat is therefore not a whole food.

> Is a steak from a feedlot steer that consumed a diet of corn, various industrial waste products, antibiotics, and hormones still a 'whole food'? I'm not so sure. The steer has itself been raised on a Western diet, and that diet has rendered its meat substantially different—in the type and amount of fat in it as well as its vitamin content—from the beef our ancestors ate. The steer's industrial upbringing has also rendered its meat so cheap that we're likely to eat more of it more often than our ancestors ever would have. This suggests yet another sense in which this beef has become an industrial food: It is designed to be eaten industrially too—as fast food.[5]

Fats and Oils: Fats and oils come from both vegetable sources and animal sources. They are fundamental for the body's structural development, mental and hormone function, insulation and protection, and the health of the nervous system, skin, hair, and cell membranes. Good fats are fortifying and necessary for the body; however, bad fats are very detrimental—disrupting organ function and clogging arteries. Hydrogenated or partially-hydrogenated vegetable oils (trans-fats) in processed food are very detrimental to health, as are saturated fats in conventionally-grown animals.

Saturated fat, commonly claimed to be unhealthy, is very good for you; it is found in fresh fruits (coconuts, nuts, avocadoes) and in animal products—all of which, in their natural forms, have sustained native peoples worldwide. Saturated fat is solid at room temperature. There is a nationwide campaign for low-fat dairy products. While the fat taken out of these conventional dairy products is probably not good for you (since fat harbors the hormones and drugs that cattle are given), organic animal fats (cream, cheese, whole milk) are much more healthful than the hydrogenated oils found in most processed foods. In trying to avoid obvious fats (whipped cream, sour cream, butter), many people still consume too many bad fats in processed foods and find themselves with excess weight and poor health. Cutting out good oils will be especially detrimental when we only eat the "hidden" and unhealthy oils in processed foods.

Good fats come from dairy products produced without hormones or antibiotics, or from cold-pressed coconut or olive oils. Cold-pressed or expeller-pressed oils are full of antioxidants and retard free-radical formation.[6] Specifically, our bodies need equal portions of omega-3 fatty acids and omega-6 fatty acids. The standard American diet is heavily weighted toward omega-6's, and most of them harmfully processed. Dairy products and coconut and olive oils were suggested above because they are all high in omega-3's. Other healthful oils exist, such as cold-pressed safflower, sunflower, and peanut oils, but they are high in omega-6's. Soybean, corn, and canola oils are not recommended by most nutritionists from whom I have gathered the other information in this book. While too complicated to explain fully here, the properties of oils are worth researching if you want to understand why there are differences. To reduce fat intake, as Americans are encouraged to do, would be like banning books because some books are worthless and filthy. That would be ridiculous! Instead, we avoid the bad ones so that we get the most benefit from the good ones—whether fats or books or whatever else it happens to be.

From *Hearth and Home*, we are told one function of dietary fat—for exercise and endurance. People that work hard physically need more fats and oils than those who are sedentary for the majority of their day.

> The body has two sources of fuel: blood sugar and fat. Sugar gives large quantities of energy for short periods of time. Fat is our endurance fuel. You must keep moving to be an efficient fat burner.[7]

Vegetables and Fruits: Vegetables and fruits are the main source of fiber in our diet (other sources are legumes, grains, nuts, and seeds), yet Americans get only one-third of the amount of fiber believed necessary for good health—and shown from history to be necessary. In 1850, people consumed three times the amount of fiber that Americans do today and had much fewer intestinal complications.[8] If disease begins in the colon, or large intestine, as many doctors believe, then fiber is very important to keep a good diet moving through your body. The best source of fiber is fresh fruits and vegetables, which have much more fiber than do enriched grain products—even those with "added fiber." Disease is bred where there is a weakened immune system, unhealthy colon, and the consumption of newfangled foods. We need fresh and old-fashioned foods to strengthen immunity, to cleanse the colon, and to counteract disease.

Seventeen percent of the American population has claimed, according to one study, that they eat zero fresh produce. Fifty percent of the population eats no vegetables except salad and potatoes (usually iceberg lettuce and French fries with ketchup).[9] Ninety percent of people eat conventionally-produced food, which includes conventionally-grown vegetables. Conventional vegetables have only twenty-five to thirty percent of the nutrients contained in organic fruit and vegetables. Diseases are increasing dramatically and the cancer rate is currently such that one in three Americans will be afflicted by it during their lifetime. All of these statistics are correlated. Most nutritionists believe that even eating the USDA-recommended servings of fresh, raw fruits and vegetables would cut the risk of degenerative diseases several-fold.

Fresh produce is cleansing and healing because it is packed with micronutrients—vitamins and minerals. Many traditional societies in temperate climates didn't have access to as many fruits and vegetables as we do today, but their animals grazed on fresh grass; hence the nutrients were transferred to the milk and meat. In our industrialized society, there are many "free-radicals" from electronics, chemicals, and air pollution that cause oxidative stress to our bodies. To counteract oxidation, we are in need of great levels of antioxidants—the elements abundant in raw foods. As stated earlier, natural color in foods indicates the presence of vitamins and minerals; hence, the fresher the produce, the better it is. Also, produce naturally contains greater amounts of useful vitamins and minerals when it hasn't been sprayed with pesticides or genetically modified—and pesticides are harmful in themselves even if they didn't harm the vitamins in vegetables. Raw foods are rich in enzymes, which are needed in an age where the nutrients in most of our foods have been depleted to some extent. Nuts and seeds contain all of the material for the emergence of life; they are truly gems packed with nutrition! People are attracted, not only to color in food, but to beauty in food—and fresh fruit or vegetable salads can be some of the most attractive, gorgeous dishes. God has given a vast variety of plant life, and for as much availability as we have in this country, there are fruits and vegetables on other continents that we don't even know about.

Some of the nutrition research executed is indeed finding the right answers, as Michel Montignac relates about high-fiber foods. However, government regulations, manufacturing practices, and consumer purchases are not at all reflecting this knowledge.

Research studies have made a convincing case for the health benefits of eating high-fiber foods, not the least of which are weight loss and long-term weight maintenance. It has been shown that eating high-fiber foods decreases blood sugar levels and lowers blood pressure, while decreasing hunger and enhancing the sensation of feeling 'full' between meals.[10]

Sugars, salt, and spices: Seasonings enhance the flavor of food, but like the rest of the food groups, they're good in their wholesome state and bad in an artificial or refined state. Refined sugars are empty calories; they provide calories for energy, and that is all they do, except for weakening the immune system and stressing the organs. Raw honey, however, is nature's only pre-digested food, and the only food that never spoils. Honey is full of antibacterial qualities and minerals and is easy to digest. Eating local honey even prevents allergies. Since bees have fed on various plants, the consumer is given just a little taste of those plants that cause allergies, and their immunity is built. Lesser-refined cane sugar such as evaporated cane juice crystals, raw sugar, sorghum, and molasses, as well as date sugar, brown rice syrup, and maple syrup, retain more minerals and are more wholesome than white sugar, but should still be used in small quantities.

Sugar in foods, especially when chocolate is involved, is a type of aphrodisiac; it makes one feel pleasure and contentment. It is not wise, however, to use the feeling that results from food as a reason to consume what is damaging to our bodies. We need to turn to the Lord with the things we are stressed about, and take responsibility for our duties, rather than turning to food as an addiction and a poor substitute for self-discipline. I am not suggesting to discard all sugar and chocolate—rather, to eat the most wholesome forms without relying on them for the feelings they induce. Certainly, there is a place for enjoying food, but when it becomes an addiction, as many unhealthy foods have the propensity to do, good things are abused.

Kick the sugary foods and invite the sensible foods, writes William Dufty. He reiterates that the quality of food is exceedingly important! Address that first, and the proper quantity naturally and easily follows. When he mentions that eating sugar cane would be less dangerous than eating refined sugar, this is because of the synergism of vitamins, minerals, and fiber in whole foods.

Kicking sugar and white flour and substituting whole grains, vegetables, and natural fruits in season is the core of any sensible natural regime. Changing the quality of your carbohydrates can change the quality of your health and life. If you eat natural food of good quality, quantity tends to take care of itself. Nobody is going to eat a half-dozen sugar beets or a whole case of sugar cane. Even if they do, it will be less dangerous than a few ounces of sugar.[11]

People take vitamins because it would be hard to acquire the same amount of a vitamin by eating ten oranges or five bunches of spinach. The same logic applies to sugar, though in the opposite way, because sugar is unhealthful. If you wouldn't eat two tall stalks of sugar cane or a bowlful of sugar beets, don't go for the concentrated version by eating refined sugar in the forms of jellied toast plus sugared cereal and sweetened fruit juice cocktail for breakfast.

Commercial table salt (refined, bleached, and iodized) has been heated and stripped of all minerals except sodium and chloride and has additives including anti-caking agents, all of which contribute to the salt building up in the human body. Real, unrefined sea salt, on the other hand, contains at least eighty essential and trace minerals which the body needs. Salt is vital to the body and has always been searched out by peoples who instinctively knew their need for salt. Refined salt today might taste similar to real salt, but it wreaks havoc on the body. Sea salt is evaporated from sea water rather than mined from mineral deposits underground. Our family has been using Celtic sea salt from Brittany on the coast of France. Celtic sea salt is beautifully colored with specks of many grays and browns and has a more delightful, mellow, and well-rounded flavor than white table salt. Again, the whitest things are not at all the best. The minerals lie with the color.

Spices and herbs—the seeds and leaves of plants—have long been valued as a medium of trade, an important economic asset, and as an exotic enhancement of food. Herbs and spices ought to have more attention than they get, for the potent, concentrated benefits that they bring to a meal in the form of antioxidants, vitamins, and minerals. A little will go a long way toward flavor as well as health. After beginning to use spices more, people can become accustomed to their delicate, complex flavors—and synthetic flavor enhancers will start to taste like what they are: artificial and lifeless. Exercise caution, however, when purchasing seasonings, for seasoning blends often contain sugar, salt, preservatives, or added flavors. Read the ingredients and buy pure spices—then learn how to use them to add excitement as well as nourishment to your food. The study of spices can be very interesting, if one tries to choose the right spices for the right food, or even the right mood. For example, Indian spices such as curry, cardamom, and turmeric are known to be very warming—perfect for seasoning a meal on a cold day. Cinnamon and parsley both aid digestion and calm the stomach. Herbs and spices are frequently used in Mediterranean cuisine, giving another reason why that diet is especially healthful.

Spices, herbs, and non-caffeinated teas are loaded with the very benefits our bodies need to combat disease. Indeed, there are many maladies in the world, but God has provided just the nutrients to prevent them. For instance, some diseases and illnesses are particularly prevented by certain vitamins: vitamin C for scurvy and vitamin B for pellagra (long known); vitamin D for influenza and vitamin B_{17} for cancer (lesser known).

There are foods that are excellent sources of each vitamin and antioxidant. Research studies continually reveal more and more healing properties of plants, and the following are just a few:

- Green tea prevents leukemia
- White tea fights obesity
- Chamomile can treat insomnia
- Blueberry leaves may heal hepatitis C
- Olive leaf can cure malaria
- Parsley is cancer-fighting
- Oregano is nature's antibiotic
- Cinnamon balances blood sugar
- Curry fights dementia
- Turmeric is a natural remedy against Alzheimer's[12]
  ...and the list could go on.

Beverages: The most neglected beverage is still the best. Water is necessary for life and comprises fifty-five to sixty percent of the human body. Water is the liquid that God has given us all over the planet and it supports life at all levels: human, plant, and animal life. Most Americans drink so many other beverages instead of water that they are acutely dehydrated and do not know it—but their organs know it, and suffer for it. A general rule is that an adult should drink at least sixty-four ounces of water daily, or eight eight-ounce glasses, and more if engaging in exercise or spending time outdoors. Liquids at meals should be consumed at room temperature or heated—not cold, and never ice cold. Cold beverages hamper the digestive juices, and some nutritionists suggest that liquid be taken a half hour before meals or after meals but never at meals. By the way, there has been refrigeration for only the last one hundred years, so people didn't regularly drink ice-cold beverages before then.

A pertinent admonition from Dr. Joseph Mercola follows. From observation, I believe he is correct; people drink hardly any water through the course of a day. From experience, I know that once a person starts to drink the recommended quota, the body will become accustomed to the new norm and become thirsty when that optimum level is not met.

Drinking eight glasses of pure water is an important foundational health principle for most people. An alarming number of Americans don't follow this guideline and are constantly dehydrated. Dehydration is subtle and most don't feel the thirst on their tongue, but their bodies are suffering—without sufficient water intake they cannot properly detoxify and aid their bodies in the elimination of wastes. Some minor symptoms of insufficient water intake are headaches, feeling tired and groggy, constipation and dry skin. If left untended, dehydration can contribute to a variety of serious health problems with blood pressure, circulation, kidney function, immune system function, and digestive disorders.[13]

Sixty percent of our body is water—and 75% of our muscles, 75% of our brain, 82% of our blood, and 25% of our bones.[14] To replenish these amounts, we need three quarts of water daily, one quart of which can be obtained from eating fresh, natural foods. So, we need roughly two more quarts of water per day, or sixty-four ounces, preferably not taken with meals and not comprised of juice, sugary, or caffeinated beverages. Processed carbohydrates—the majority of the American diet—are starchy, contain very little water, and are loaded with sodium, which is dehydrating. People eating those foods will need to drink more than two quarts of water to stay hydrated because their food is definitely not providing the third quart.

Thirst is a signal of *dehydration*, not a signal for when our body needs more water. We do need it when it we are thirsty, of course, especially after strenuous exercise or time out in the sun; but we need it long before we "feel" it. While dehydration contributes to countless symptoms and diseases, hydration helps skin clarity, circulation and digestion, and prevents disease.

What most people drink when they are thirsty actually dehydrates the body and has the reverse effect that water does. Coffee and other caffeinated drinks are diuretics, removing fluids from the body. For every cup of caffeinated beverage consumed, two cups of water should be consumed to counteract the dehydration. Green, black, white, and red teas are exceptionally high in antioxidants and are more beneficial than coffee, especially in their decaffeinated forms. Most herbal teas (herbal tisanes) don't contain caffeine and are a good alternative choice to coffee, hot cocoa, or caffeinated tea.

At the risk of censuring the favorite addiction of millions worldwide, but with the desire to warn people that they drink to their own impairment, I'd like to make a further note about coffee. Caffeine, which many people get from a multi-daily dose of coffee, is "a very powerful drug," as Dr. Mercola calls it—a drug which depletes our B vitamins vital for energy, fosters many health disorders, and contributes to low birth weight in babies of mothers who intake caffeine while pregnant. Coffee is a "substance which places an enormous metabolic burden on your body and offers no nutritional value at all." Dr. Mercola continues, in just one of countless treatises on the dangers of caffeine, "Just like with most drugs, there are perceived benefits—and then there are the side effects which often render the "cure" worse than the disease."[15]

Along with the delivery of purportedly fine taste or extra energy for which most people drink coffee, the liquid delivers a whole host of problems right into your bloodstream. Is coffee necessary enough that you have to fuel your addiction and drink to your injury—no, I didn't mean energy—in order to have that enjoyable taste in your mouth? Also, caffeine is not the only undesirable factor in coffee, so even decaffeinated coffee poses numerous problems to the body. I hope you will consider doing enough research so that you are confident about the wisdom of the choice you have made to drink or not to drink coffee. (If you do decide to drink it, at least use organic coffee and flavor it with real sugar and real cream.) God created our bodies to depend on food; He did not create our bodies to depend upon drugs.

Most processed beverages, such as sodas and sport drinks, are full of sugar, artificial colors, artificial flavors, and other chemicals. They are harmful for the reasons already discussed regarding sugars and artificial additives. Soda pulls calcium from the bones and is therefore especially injurious to children in their growing years and women in their middle age. Caffeine in cold drinks is more potent than caffeine in hot drinks. Some sodas have at least seventy artificial flavors and preservatives in them according to one study, not to mention high fructose corn syrup, and the average American drinks 600 sodas per year.[16] If a beverage must be had, purchase or make one with pure, simple ingredients. Lemonade, for instance, can be made with water, lemon juice, and honey rather than canned powders that are mostly artificial. For a punch or soda for a special occasion, you can purchase or make beverages with plain carbonated water mixed with unsweetened fruit juice.

Popular energy drinks with sugar, caffeine, alcohol, and other drugs in them are quite awful, with no redeeming value at all. Each of those ingredients is harmful and addictive and should be avoided. Energy drinks cause the heart to race, and consumption of drinks containing active drug ingredients has been linked to violence and sudden deaths. There is no good substitute for sleep and good food, both of which God has prescribed in His Word. People who try to make their own sources of high-dose energy will end up paying for it in other ways. For true, life-giving energy, look for or make your own vegetable and fruit juices with no added sugar or high fructose corn syrup in them. Fresh juices have only healthful properties—a far cry from energy drinks and their only-destructive properties.

We used to mix together artificial fruit drinks frequently for lunch when I was young. I thought it was just a fun alternative to juice. Actually, I remember being a little skeptical of the blue and green colors—not exactly the colors of fruit! Well, with the entire cup of sugar per jug, and artificial colors and flavors, I will not go anywhere near it now. It is definitely not fruit juice—not even a hint.

Alcohol—wine and beer—is so controversial in terms of health as well as religious preferences, that I hesitate to make any firm judgments. Biblically, the pleasurable drinking of alcohol seems to be accepted, yet there are strong cautions against its abuse. It should be agreed that alcoholic drinks have much potential for damage in the brain and body when used to excess, and potential for birth defects when used at all by child-bearing women. From my research, it seems possible that any benefits claimed from red wine particularly, such as bioflavanoids or antiviral and anti-inflammatory properties, could be received from alternative sources. Some medical doctors believe that alcohol raises the blood pressure, suppresses the nervous and immune systems, blocks absorption of nutrients, and injures the organs.[17] Any substance that is harmful in a large quantity and highly addictive, like alcohol is, should have much caution and consideration attached to its use. Drinks with high alcohol content, such as hard liquor, are far more detrimental to the body than is wine. Since I have been interested in the historical aspects of diet, it is of note that traditional societies have usually used fermented drinks of various kinds. Certainly, intoxicating alcohol has long been produced, as the Genesis record indicates. Also, slight fermentation was one historic way of preserving water and juice for voyages or for aiding digestion.

Regardless of the decision people come to regarding energy drinks and alcohol, taste buds need to be retrained to love water and natural drinks, for those will supply all of the things that our bodies truly need. Foods, drinks, drugs, and other stimulants that abruptly alter our bodies, whether for sleep, energy, excitement, alertness, or whatever else, are questionable. Christians should be steadfast and constant in lifestyle, which is contrary to the felt-need to vacillate between feeling drowsy, feeling great, needing to stay awake, or needing to fall asleep. The nutrients we need to sleep well, and then to have energy throughout the next day, are amply found in wholesome food and drinks.

I should note that the chemicals and artificial ingredients in foods have been developed that way for a reason. Usually the natural compound of something (something that gives us energy, or something that gives us a certain flavor) is studied and either multiplied or mimicked with concentrated chemical compounds. The form God created is used, then, to some extent, but the end product is totally different and artificial. Since, of course, man cannot create anything new, he has to use or alter what is already made by God.

Disobedience often stems from the desire to have something that *can* be good, outside of or before the time or place that God has designed it to be. Additionally, sin often stems from a desire to have more of something than is sufficient and prudent for us. Leisure can be a special reward, but to spend our whole lives in that way would mean neglecting many of God's commands for diligence and labor. Rich food might be used on celebratory occasions, but to eat in this way all the time would be foolish and extravagant.

To go back to my point, artificial foods and chemical stimulants give more of any given substance than we were meant to have at one time. What good food will provide gradually and consistently, drugs provide in a rush. Stimulants give results all at once rather than our having to wait patiently and exercise discipline. Chemicals change our bodies hastily; and hastening toward unwise things is far from a Christian virtue.

Chapter Twenty

Battle for the Balance

"To win a major war, you must first identify and locate the enemy."[1]
—Dr. Don Colbert

GOD MADE OUR bodies to be resilient and strong, but also intricate and delicate. Our bodies perform outstandingly with the proper fuel and care, but start to have unseemly problems when the proper fuel and care is replaced by carelessness. Like an old-fashioned set of scales, the kind of input that our body gets will have the most weight—the most influence—on our health.

Free-radicals attack our cells and antioxidants fortify our cells; which will you allow into your body? The human body will only last so long. Will you strengthen it for its task or let it become weak through neglect? Will you invest in your health or tear it down with your hands (and mouth)? Basically, the quality and kinds of food that we eat make all the difference for good or ill. We are surrounded and assailed daily by toxins, but we can fight against them by the foods we eat. We know that our bodies wear out as they age, but we can anticipate that process by building them up nutritionally at the same time.

Preliminary to Dr. Colbert's following illustration of the players in a battle is the idea that there is a war going on. Christians are living on a battlefield and are constantly in a battle—a battle for good or evil, spiritually, and a battle for health or harm, physically.

To win a major war, you must first identify and locate the enemy. The number one adversary we face is free radicals...Free radicals are the bad guys and antioxidants are the good guys. Unfortunately, we have left the gates open to the enemy soldiers and have not employed the forces to defeat them.[2]

A battle is comprised of the onslaught of opposing forces. The delicate balance of our health is certainly an instance of opposing forces fighting to win. Which will have the victory? Will we passively allow the onslaught of the effects of sin (sickness, disease, and people destroying and meddling with God's world) to be victorious? On the other hand, will we actively seek the aggressive task of battling sin (and sin's effects in our health and diet) with the wisdom from His Word and with true dominion work whereby people understand, love, restore and cultivate His creation? As for me, I want to be on the right side of the battle—the same side as God—where His Word is honored and where He is bringing the chaotic, unrighteous world into subjection to Him. The Christians I talk to want to be on God's side, too, and many of them are making the effort to honor Him in their diets. That is the big picture of the battle that is raging concerning our bodies.

Another issue to address is how our bodies handle different inputs, such as free-radicals and antioxidants, either being attacked by them or attacking them. Free-radicals and antioxidants attack each other, so we obviously need more of the "good guys," using them strategically. To tie this back to the previous paragraph, antioxidants come straight from God's creation, whereas free-radicals are largely the work of man (coming from chemicals, over-processing of food and oils, and environmental hazards.) These ideas do not imply that we should live in a place untouched by man. God commands mankind to cultivate the earth for His glory. However, we do need a healthful diet to counteract many of the things we are exposed to—fuels and fumes in the air, electrical currents, etc.

Dr. Bruce Fife in *The Coconut Oil Miracle* explains the difference between free radicals, linked to over sixty diseases, and antioxidants, our only protection from disease. As I said before and will say again, there are some astute doctors who are also teachers. These are the men and women from whom we need to learn. Acquire professional advice from people who understand the battle like Dr. Fife portrays it here:

Once a molecule becomes a radical, its physical and chemical properties are permanently changed. When this molecule is part of a living cell, it affects the function of the entire cell. Free radicals can attack our cells, literally ripping their protective membranes apart...The more free radicals attack our cells, the greater the damage and the greater the potential for serious destruction to vital organs, joints, and bodily systems....We are exposed to free radicals from the pollutants in the air we breathe and from the chemical additives and toxins in the foods we eat and drink.[3]

Free radicals tear, attack, and pollute. Antioxidants heal, protect, and cleanse. Renegade molecules are not what we want in our bodies; we want our bodies to be under subjection. Notice where Dr. Fife says we are exposed to free radicals. To be on the offensive, we need adequate antioxidants.

> The only way to stop a free radical is with an antioxidant. Antioxidants are molecules that neutralize free radicals, making them harmless...We can get antioxidants in fresh fruits and vegetables, but most people don't eat enough of these to provide significant protection.[4]

The author goes on to show why coconut oil, truly a remarkable oil, is loaded with antioxidants, and being a healthy saturated fat, these properties remain stable on the shelf and accessible to the body once ingested. He makes distinct mention of this property of coconut oil because it is completely opposite of most vegetable oils which are, instead, major sources of free-radicals.

Carbohydrates are another thing which, depending on their quality, will either strengthen or weaken the body. We need energy, but energy isn't neutral. Energy fights on one side of the battle or the other. Refined carbohydrates provide quick, fleeting energy that leaves behind a trail of damage and continually requires more of the same fuel. Wholesome carbohydrates provide deep, enduring energy so there is less need for rapid replenishment and no damage suffered.

Dr. Ray Strand and Bill Ewing's words clarify the important but potentially adverse place of carbohydrates in our diets. You should be thinking *quality* and *quantity* as you read this! "Roller-coaster ride" is a fitting image.

> Carbohydrates provide the fuel that the body and the brain desire, and good carbohydrates contain the vitamins, minerals, and antioxidants that our bodies need. We have to learn, however, that there are good carbohydrates and there are bad carbohydrates. The root issue is the fact that certain carbohydrates are converted unnaturally fast into blood sugar within our bodies. When these foods are consumed on a regular basis, the body is set on a roller-coaster ride of rising and falling blood-sugar levels that God never designed it to cope with—and the results are often deadly.[5]

In a sense, food is either living or dead. Food is either fresh and natural or it has been processed and changed so much it little resembles the original plant or animal. Within the sovereignty of God, food contributes either to our life or to our death. Food either hurts us or helps us, making our life one of sluggishness or making it full of vitality.

Dr. Don Colbert has explained that we have trillions of cells that are replaced every year. What we feed them has a huge impact on whether our bodies become stronger or weaker, and whether health is being gained or lost. He says that living foods contain essential nutrients and enzymes, but that most of the American diet is comprised of foods that have been cooked and overcooked, even "cooked to death." Consequently, a diet of fifty percent raw food is a good measure.[6] In *What You Don't Know May Be Killing You,* he outlines the process that takes place when we eat enzyme-depleted food. When there is no life in the food eaten, the body draws life from itself—and this, as it would be expected, leads to degeneration of every kind. Life is necessary for regeneration. Below is a brief excerpt:

> As your cells die and are replaced, the new cells are totally dependent on the building materials available...When food is cooked until the enzymes have been lost, our bodies are forced to draw upon our metabolic enzymes—the raw materials and the spark that rebuilds our bodies...

> Note carefully this important principle: If we eat more raw, uncooked foods, our bodies will not need to expend their valuable metabolic enzymes to make digestive enzymes.[7]

Food may be placed into the following two categories: food that manufactures free-radicals in your body and food that manufactures antioxidants for your body. One kind invests in your bodily health; the other is a drain on your asset of health. Manmade food renders a body that looks like it was tampered with by sinful man; God-created food renders a body that looks like it was made by an all-wise God. Our bodies *are* made by God, whether a person believes it or not, so we can expect that our bodies will operate best on the fuel He designed.

Dr. Ben Lerner, in *Body by God,* divides food into "Food by Man" and "Food by God." He explains that Food by God is naturally and easily digested and dispensed to the cells, where its vital nutrients can be used directly. Food by Man, on the other hand, cannot be digested easily, instead building up in the body, clogging the organs, and leaving the cells with no vital replenishment. Food with life in it sustains life, but lifeless food attacks life—in the form of malady and disease.

> Food by God is smart food. When you eat Food by God, such as an apple or a carrot, it knows what to do inside the BBG [Body by God], and the intelligent BBG knows what to do with it...

Food by Man is created by man and so does not contain any of God's intelligence. Therefore, it does not know what to do in the BBG, and the BBG has no idea what to do with it.[8]

Those few sentences are very striking. Some food knows what to do in the body, and other food products do not. When food can't nourish you, it ends up accumulating in other ways and then eventually affecting health. The parts of food products that are not real food (such as MSG or hydrogenated oil) cannot act like food so they act in other ways—causing headaches, heart disease, and more.

Speaking of food knowing what to do in the body, did you know that there seem to be characteristics in God's foods that seem to match the appearance of organs that they particularly nourish? Some people have noticed nutritional associations between walnuts and the human brain, sliced carrots and eyes, tomatoes and the heart, onions and bodily cells, sweet potatoes and the pancreas, avocadoes and figs and reproductive organs, celery stalks and bones, kidney beans and kidneys, and more.

Returning to a previous point, a beef cow is an example of a food that can be either a free-radical factory or antioxidant factory, depending upon several things. If a cow is raised on grass during the summer and a little grain in the fall when grasses go to seed, it is eating what God designed it to eat. If you harvest it during autumn, preserve it for winter, and grill it for your family, you are eating God-created food. However, if a cow was raised under artificial light during the winter, fed on high-fructose corn, and injected with antibiotics to be kept alive amidst filthy conditions, it is maturing in a manmade environment. If the beef is ground up, blended with more high-fructose corn in the form of syrup, loaded with preservatives, and packaged into jerky strips, it is man-altered food. Now, of course, we need to combine ingredients and we need to cook food; combining or cooking is not the issue. Food is "manmade" if its very nature is changed. Cows were not made to eat corn syrup, but green grass and hay. Artificial preservatives, such as in packaged beef jerky, keep meat from spoiling when it otherwise would. However, if beef steak is frozen, it is virtually the same when it is thawed out.

Man-altered foods use things which God did not put together. God made fruit to be sweet and colorful and appealing to us, full of vitamins and fiber and water. Most conventional fruit spreads, though, add white sugar and artificial coloring to the fruit. While fruit itself is entirely usable to our bodies, we don't need the extra sugar and color found in most jams. Our bodies cannot use excess sugar and artificial color to promote vitality, so our bodies convert those ingredients into other things, such as excess fat or hyperactivity. In biblical times, women ground grain to make bread and combined ingredients to make stews; however, they didn't separate the germ and bran from the wheat kernel, and they didn't add poisonous flavor enhancers like MSG to their soups.

Man tries to add or take away from God's foods, and ends up with substances to which our bodies react. Manmade foods weaken and imbalance our body's strong but delicate composition when what we need is balance and proper growth.

The men in my family have done business brokerage for three generations. My grandfather started in his seventies, my father in his forties, and my brother in his teen years. Having worked for both my dad and brother, and after years of hearing them talk about the industry and about their particular engagements, I find the profession fascinating and enjoy finding object lessons from the things spoken about. I find it interesting that business terminology can apply to many different things, including nutrition. For instance, the industry term for transactions is "mergers and acquisitions," so when my brother got married, we said that he was making an acquisition and merging their two lives.

One major business sector with which my family members have dealt is manufacturing and distribution. In relation to nutrition, I like to think of our bodies as manufacturers and distributors. We manufacture enzymes and cells in our blood and tissue. Children, especially, do this in their growing years. Our bodies are distributors of information through our brain and nervous systems, and distributors of nutrients through our blood and digestive systems. We take in food and distribute it to the parts of our body, and we manufacture cells to replace old ones. This manufacturing and distribution is a constant process, with most of the fuel being taken in and distributed during the day, and most of the rebuilding or manufacturing happening while we sleep.

What makes a business a unique kind of possession or entity (generally unlike a house or vehicle) is the fact that it is *liquid*—the value is constantly being adjusted by the inflow and outflow of money and products or services. Our bodies are similar; they are always being affected by the food we put in them and by the health that is being either fortified or diminished as a result.

The life of a business is represented by its balance sheets and profit/loss statements, and these standards can be applied to our health as well. The health of our bodies is like a balance sheet; food is either an asset or a liability, and the bottom line shows which one you have in the greater amount. The more liabilities accumulated, the more your body will be in debt, losing more nutrients than it takes in, becoming weakened, and becoming answerable to its creditor—sickness. The more assets, or wholesome nutritious food that you have, the more your body will be enriched by consuming the food it should have and by becoming stronger. Will your next meal be an asset or a liability to the health balance of your body?

Profit and loss statements are likewise applicable, except that the commodities concerned are healthy cells and nutrients rather than dollars and cents. Your body is either gaining or losing nutrients, and the bottom line is whether or not the levels are reaching into the red (danger) zone. So many toxins attack our immune systems that we need more nutrients than ever to counteract the toxins, lest our immune systems become compromised. We need more input of nutrients to provide for the inevitable output. Some things always *expend* our bodies—aging, accidents, viruses, and chemical exposure, to name a few things. We need to seek the things—food, supplements, exercise, and a healthy environment—that will *invest* in our bodies.

Any wise business person knows that you need more income than expenses to survive—in fact, a lot more in order to invest the profit in greater endeavors and grow the company into the future. Let us be wise stewards of our bodies, building them up and keeping them in an advantageous condition for God's service.

We have considered the two sides in the battle for our health, we have looked at the opposition of free-radicals and antioxidants, and we have discussed food being either an asset or a liability. Something else to consider is not only eating good, profitable food, but doing it in balanced proportions.

Healthfulness demands a balance of alkaline-producing and acid-producing foods. Plans exist to shape diets with a proper amount of each, since American diets tend to be very acid-producing and in need of food input that causes alkaline-production. It is best to eat from sixty to seventy-five percent alkaline-producing foods, and from twenty-five to forty percent acid-producing foods. Perhaps you can guess—processed carbohydrates are highly acid-producing, and fruits and vegetables are alkaline-producing! The standard American diet is forever a culprit, whether it imbalances the acid-alkaline ratio, heightens blood sugar to unhealthy levels, imbalances the proper omega-3 and omega-6 ratio, or depletes vitamin and mineral levels.

Different health and diet programs, including very good ones that suggest eating whole, natural foods, will give recommendations for varying proportions of various nutrients, or suggest what to eat at certain times. Skipping breakfast and eating a heavy dinner will lead to weight gain; it is best to have more evenly-proportioned meals. In fact, eating a large breakfast and smaller evening meal most corresponds to the needful burning of calories. People wanting to lose weight might eat more proteins and low-glycemic carbohydrates, as *The French Diet* recommends. People that are physically active will need more fats that the less active. *Body by God* suggests that eating carbohydrates provides energy for the morning, and that eating protein builds and restores muscles in the evening. *Dr. Mercola's Total Health Program* prescribes eating plans for body types that lean toward needing protein versus body types needing carbohydrates—and how to know which one you are.

All of these suggestions are dependent on your health, your metabolic type, and your activity level. Generally, nutritionists recommend that proteins and starches are combined with vegetables, not with each other in a heavy meal of fifty percent protein and fifty percent starchy carbohydrates. It is recommended that fruit is more digestible when eaten alone, except if one is prone to high blood sugar. Paying attention to the balance of food groups in your diet, and the combinations at any given meal, can be very beneficial as you heed the affect of your diet on energy levels and digestion.

Given the bold distinctions and contrasts discussed in this chapter and others, I want to clarify that categories of foods and bodily input are not always *black and white*. While principles can be applied in choosing good food—indeed, the subject of this book—I do not intend to imply that unhealthy foods have absolutely no value. Nor do I want to condemn those foods or the people eating them. Certainly, many people have long eaten the popular foods produced by American technology, and even persons concerned about nutrition have occasion to eat those foods. What I intend to get across to the reader is that there are differences in how food is produced and the effect it has on our bodies. While conventionally-produced food products do have an amount of value—since they do feed and fill us—they doubtlessly contain harmful substances and have gone through awful processes. While that is food to an extent, it is not *pure* food. My tenet is that pure, wholesome food nourishes, sustains, and heals while impure, adulterated food brings slow damage along with its lessened merit.

There are not always only two obvious categories of healthful versus harmful foods. Books such as *Nourishing Traditions* and *Patient, Heal Thyself* give three or four increments of edibility of food and list foods that are moderately healthy and moderately unhealthy, as well as hurtful foods and healing foods. It takes wisdom and grace to balance the food choices we make with the many other social demands that we have—such as thankfulness for hospitality and flexibility in travel. While it is good to have a strong standard and to understand our food and differences thereof, nothing should be held above ours or anyone else's heads as an ultimate standard. God's Word is the only true standard for conduct and the spiritual battle is the only battle that reaches into eternity—and while His Word commands us to care for our earthly temples, Scripture also says that we are not to judge another person's meat and drink. God's kingdom does not consist in meat and drink but in righteousness, grace, and peace.

That being said, a physical and ideological battle *is* seething as we choose what to eat and as food makes its way into and through our bodies. We need to be on the wise side of the conflict, aiding our bodies and working alongside God in His restoration of all creation. While God does not promise success in our earthly life, He promises ultimate victory for those who live by faith in Him. I want to be working toward vitality and victory, not sickness and surrender. What about you?

Chapter Twenty-one

Charts for Comparison

"High-tech tomatoes. Mysterious milk. Supersquash. Are we
supposed to eat this stuff? Or is it going to eat us?"[1]

—Annita Manning

ONLY TEN PERCENT of Americans buy what can be considered as healthful groceries.[2] The following charts show what is healthful and what is definitely not healthful. Pay close attention to the complexity and unwholesomeness of the ingredients in the left column, and the simplicity and wholeness of the ingredients in the right column. These charts are far from comprehensive, but should provide helpful guidelines.

	Ingredients and Methods Commonly Used in Conventional Manufacturing:	Ingredients and Methods Commonly Used in Organic or Natural Manufacturing:
Wheat Snack Crackers	Enriched flour, partially hydrogenated soybean oil, whole grain wheat flour, sugar, defatted wheat germ, cornstarch, malt syrup, high fructose corn syrup, salt, monoglycerides, leavening, natural flavor, caramel color, soy lecithin, sodium sulfite.	Organic unbleached flour, organic buttermilk, organic expeller pressed safflower oil, organic stone ground whole wheat flour, organic evaporated cane juice, brown rice syrup, organic corn meal, organic quinoa, organic flax meal, wheat germ, water, sea salt, baking soda, turmeric.

Continued

	Ingredients and Methods Commonly Used in Conventional Manufacturing:	Ingredients and Methods Commonly Used in Organic or Natural Manufacturing:
Granola Bars	Popular brands contain several kinds of sweeteners; one brand has sugar, brown sugar syrup, honey, *and* high fructose corn syrup. Bars are usually made with soy products, hydrogenated soybean oil, and synthetic emulsifiers. "Natural and artificial flavors" are a mask for virtually anything approved for use in flavoring food.	Organic brands might contain several kinds of natural sugars: brown rice syrup, evaporated cane juice, and organic molasses. The oil in organic bars is usually expeller-pressed. The oat fiber in one type of organic bar gave it five times the amount of fiber as its conventional counterpart.
Tortillas	Enriched bleached flour, water, partially hydrogenated vegetable oil, glycerin, corn syrup solids, salt, baking powder (with aluminum sulfate), potassium sorbate, monosodium phosphate, phosphoric acid, calcium propionate, sodium acid pyrphosphate, monoglycerides, fumaric acid.	Organic whole wheat flour, organic wheat flour, organic spelt flour, water, organic extra virgin olive oil or organic palm oil, organic soy fiber, apple cider vinegar, organic honey, organic raisin puree, baking powder (aluminum-free), sea salt, organic guar gum, ascorbic acid (Vitamin C).
Roasting Chicken	High in unhealthy saturated fat from feeding on grain-based feed and animal parts. Grown in indoor confinement housing and contaminated by waste and its particles in the air. Meat is dry and mushy and nine percent of its weight is said to be fecal sludge. The air exchange in confinement houses is far from clean, but the chickens are kept moving through until slaughter. Birds, upon butchering, receive chlorine baths to kill bacteria.	Lower and healthier fat than conventional chickens because of exercise and diet of grass and insects. Grown in coops or pens outside, with access to fresh air; moved often to clean paddocks. Chlorophyll in green diets benefits our bodies. Meat is solid yet moist. "When animals are fed a high-energy, low vitamin-mineral diet, they tend to have more saturated fat (cholesterol) in their meat, milk, or eggs, just like people. When these same animals consume a large portion of green material, the saturated fat of their animal proteins diminishes."[3]

	Ingredients and Methods Commonly Used in Conventional Manufacturing:	Ingredients and Methods Commonly Used in Organic or Natural Manufacturing:
Whole Milk	Confined cows average only 1.8 lactations (periods of milk production) in their lifetime but produce 20,000 pounds of milk annually. With this taxation on their systems, they become weak and sickly before they are butchered. Pesticides from feed and residue from injected hormones and antibiotics are found in milk when tested. Pasteurization and homogenization (the latter patented in 1901) are destructive to natural enzymes and vitamins in milk. Raw milk was consumed for millennia, yet pasteurization is said to be absolutely necessary. Around 1995, whole milk consumption per capita was eighty pounds (largely replaced by low-fat milk), down from 168 pounds in 1975; yet more Americans are overweight than ever.[4]	Pasture-fed cows average 8-10 lactations in their lifetime and can produce 400 pounds of milk annually throughout their lifetime. The cows are healthy; the milk is free of hormones and pesticides (in organic milk). The milk is full of good fats and naturally occurring vitamins if the cows have been fed on green grass outdoors. If it's hard to find raw milk, at least try to purchase organic milk produced without hormones, antibiotics, or confinement. The cows are healthier, and the milk will be, too.
Eggs	Low nutrients and very low omega-3 fatty acids; produced in and affected by the same filthy environment as the poultry described above.	Good source of high concentration of omega-3 fatty acids; grass-fed chickens convert vitamins into the eggs they produce.
Meat Franks	Pork, mechanically separated turkey, water, corn syrup, salt, partially hydrolyzed beef stock, dextrose, autolyzed yeast, potassium lactate, sodium phosphates, sodium lactate, sodium erythobate, sodium diacetate, sodium nitrate, flavorings, ascorbic acid, extractives of paprika.	Organic beef, water, sea salt, celery juice, lactic acid starter culture, organic raw sugar, organic onion powder, organic paprika, ground mustard, pepper, garlic, nutmeg, and coriander.
Yogurt	Milk, strawberries, natural and artificial flavors, live cultures, cornstarch, gluten, aspartame, fructose, pectin, gelatin, carmine.	Organic whole milk, organic cream, organic strawberries, organic sugar, beet juice concentrate, natural vanilla, live active probiotic cultures.

	Ingredients and Methods Commonly Used in Conventional Manufacturing:	Ingredients and Methods Commonly Used in Organic or Natural Manufacturing:
Potatoes	Genetically modified potatoes are heavily sprayed with pesticides during maturation and with sprout inhibitors after harvest. Most of the pesticides are retained in the skin.	No pesticides or herbicides or anti-sprouting sprays. The skin, pesticide-free, is the most mineral- and fiber-rich part of an organic potato.
Spaghetti Sauce	Tomatoes, diced tomatoes, corn syrup, soybean oil, salt; spices, dehydrated garlic, dehydrated onion, dehydrated parsley, citric acid, natural flavors [vague—includes any substance approved for food use.]	Vine-ripened tomatoes, diced tomatoes, tomato puree, onions, garlic, pure Italian extra virgin olive oil, salt, fresh garlic, fresh basil, fresh parsley, honey. [Spices are all specified; nothing is hidden.]
Canned Vegetable Soup	Beef stock, potatoes, carrots, tomato puree, green beans, water, peas, cornstarch, rehydrated onions, modified corn, salt, yeast extract, hydrolyzed wheat gluten, soy protein, partially hydrogenated vegetable oil, monosodium glutamate, spice extract, caramel color, chicken flavor.	Filtered water, organic tomatoes, organic carrots, organic kidney beans, organic potatoes, organic celery, organic leeks, organic peas, organic semolina flour, organic spinach, sea salt, organic sunflower oil, organic garlic, organic cornstarch, black pepper.
Packaged Lettuce	Thin, moist leaves of lettuce harbor pesticides more than other produce does. Preservatives sprayed on pre-packaged lettuce can be tasted prior to dressing.	Organic lettuce does not last as long as treated lettuce, but is pure and clean, with no residual spray either inside the leaves or on the leaves.
Pie Filling	Apples, high fructose corn syrup, water, corn syrup, food starch-modified, natural flavor, spices, erythorbic acid.	Unpeeled apple slices, sugar, cornstarch, xanthan gum, spices.
Coconut Pudding	Sugar, modified food starch, coconut, artificial flavor, disodium phosphate, tetrasodium pyrophosphate, Yellow 5, Yellow 6, sodium metabisulfite, BHA.	Organic cane sugar, organic coconut, organic cornstarch, organic pumpkin powder, organic sea salt, organic vanilla.
Mayonnaise	Canola or soybean oil, water, eggs, distilled vinegar, lemon juice concentrate, salt, sugar, dried onion, dried garlic, paprika, natural flavor, calcium disodium EDTA.	Expeller pressed safflower oil, apple cider vinegar, filtered water, salt, egg whites, dehydrated cane juice, onion, garlic, paprika, lemon juice, honey.

	Ingredients and Methods Commonly Used in Conventional Manufacturing:	Ingredients and Methods Commonly Used in Organic or Natural Manufacturing:
Salad Dressing	Soybean oil, water, vinegar, sugar, salt, garlic juice, natural buttermilk flavor, phosphoric acid, polysorbate 60, spice, dried parsley, lemon juice concentrate, disodium inosinate, disodium guanylate, calcium disodium EDTA, monosodium glutamate, natural and artificial flavor.	Sunflower oil, water, apple cider vinegar, buttermilk powder, cane sugar, sea salt, onions, carrot powder, celery seed, garlic, chives, parsley, xanthan gum.
Peanut Butter	Peanuts, corn syrup, sugar, molasses, hydrogenated vegetable oils, soy protein, salt, pyridoxine hydrochloride, ferric orthophosphate, copper sulfate.	Organic dry roasted peanuts, sea salt.
Chocolate Syrup	High fructose corn syrup, milk chocolate, water, corn syrup, cornstarch, partially hydrogenated soybean oil, sweetened condensed milk, sugar, whey, soy lecithin, cocoa, mono and diglycerides, disodium phosphate, sodium citrate, artificial vanillin flavor, potassium sorbate (preservative), salt, polysorbate 60.	Organic cane sugar, water, organic cocoa, organic coconut oil, organic vanilla extract, xanthan gum.
Chocolate Cookies	Enriched flour, sugar, hydrogenated vegetable oil, cocoa, high fructose corn syrup, baking soda, salt, soy lecithin, artificial vanillin flavor, Blue 2, Yellow 6, Red 40.	Organic wheat flour, organic sugar, organic palm oil, organic chocolate chips, organic oats, organic vanilla, baking soda, salt.
Root Beer	Carbonated water, high fructose corn syrup, caramel color, sodium benzoate, natural and artificial flavors.	Sparkling filtered water; molasses; evaporated cane juice; caramel color; wintergreen, birch, anise, sassafras, nutmeg, licorice, sarsaparilla, and Tahitian vanilla extracts; phosphoric acid.

Following are a few comments about food additives, to provoke thought; the information available is endless and this only uncovers the surface. The left column describes food that has been altered in some way or several ways; the right column describes food in its original or nearly original state. Again, by 'altered' I don't mean blending or combining, but processes such as hydrogenating or bleaching. By 'natural,' I don't mean food untouched by man, but food that has been cooked or extracted simply and unobtrusively.

Some Attributes of Processed or Artificial Food Products:	Some Attributes of Pure and Wholesome Food Products:
Cold Cereal	*Cooked Grain*
Most nutrients destroyed; processing hampers digestibility; refined carbohydrates raise blood sugar as much as, or more than, white sugar. "Slurried and extruded at high temperatures and pressures."[5] Very expensive for its weight, and low nutrient value! Usually high in sugar, colorings, hydrogenated oils, preservatives, and other additives. It has been argued that there is more nutrition in the box itself than in the cereal. (No wonder my mom used to call packaged, instant oatmeal "cardboard mush"! Now, she likes oatmeal made from scratch at home.)	Cooked grains have nourished the whole world in their whole form since the beginning of history. Cooked grains contain all of the nutrients of the kernels/berries, including vitamins, minerals and fiber. If soaked before cooking, the nutrients are even more accessible to the body in digestion.
White Rice	*Brown Rice*
Polished rice causes disease, including beriberi—a disease of the nervous system from a deficiency of B vitamins, especially thiamine. With food of deficient nutrient value, such as white rice, the body uses previously eaten nutrients to digest the present meal, such as white rice; the overall result is a depletion of nutrients, not a gain. White rice drains your health and energy, instead of sustaining your life. Undersupply of B vitamins can lead to depression, but many people are on drugs to treat depression, covering it up and causing side affects rather than finding the real problem: lack of whole grains and other whole foods.	Rich in B vitamins, which boost morale. "If your system is deprived of even a single food chemical, your mental state may suffer...Mental alertness, then, like emotional stability, serenity, an even and pleasant disposition, and a zest for living have all been shown to suffer when dietary intake of thiamine is low."[6] Brown rice is flavorful on its own, with no need for seasonings or sauces. There are gourmet organic varieties available, or blends of brown rice and wild rice. Brown jasmine rice has all the fragrance of jasmine rice and all the nutrients of brown rice.
Margarine	*Butter*
Margarine is artificially hydrogenated, colored, and flavored, is loaded with trans-fats, blocks arteries, and inhibits digestion. In its altered molecular composition, margarine acts similar to butter in the kitchen, but in the body has a negative affect on digestion—the very opposite of butter. Margarine has often been called "plastic" and rightly so, since both are made from molecularly-altered oil and neither is very digestible.	If from organic, grass-fed cattle, butter is full of vitamins (from the green grass) and healthy saturated fat. Countless studies show, and history proves, that people thrive on butter; healthy butter does not cause weight gain. Any butter helps the absorption of other foods during digestion and is far better than margarine, yet organic butter is much better for you than butter from hormone-injected, grain-fed cows.

Some Attributes of Processed or Artificial Food Products:	Some Attributes of Pure and Wholesome Food Products:
Hydrogenated or Partially-hydrogenated Vegetable Oil	*Cold-pressed Olive Oil*
"Manmade molecules" that are a "nutritional disaster."[7] Hydrogenated oil was invented in 1901; by 1921, it was strongly linked to heart disease, which had recently become the leading cause of death in the United States. Hydrogenation turns liquids into solids using high heat, starch, and chemical and metal emulsifiers.

If soybeans and corn are used to fatten cattle, then why are soybean and corn oil popularly used and recommended for human "health" and weight management? These oils contribute to unneeded body fat, and soy oil—comprising much of "vegetable" oil—damages the thyroid, leading to many other ailments.

"Trans-fats are found only in foods that have been altered and conform neither to the primitive diet nor to the intent of our Maker."[8]

"Hydrogenated oil is a product of technology and may be the most destructive food additive currently in common use."[9] | Olive oil is a healthy oil mentioned in the Bible; it is high in omega-3 fatty acids; it protects the heart and prevents disease (and is minimally processed).

We need fats in our diet, but not the kind that accumulate around the waist. Olive oil, a kind of oil that our body capably metabolizes, supports our bodily systems in the best way possible.

Eating high-omega-3 oils will help to balance the proportion of omega-6 and omega-3 oils for our bodies. It is easy enough to get omega-6 oils from grains and other foods; we need to concentrate on getting omega-3's from the fats we consume.

We make sure to put the proper kind of oil in our vehicles; how very much more important are proper oils for the function of our bodies! |
| *White Vinegar* | *Apple Cider Vinegar* |
| White vinegar is distilled and has absolutely zero health value. Harsh solvents are used in the manufacturing. White vinegar is great for natural house-cleaning, though! | Wonderful health benefits for weight loss, settling the stomach, and killing bad bacteria internally or externally. It flushes impurities and relieves pain.

Raw organic apple cider vinegar "contains the amazing 'mother of vinegar' which occurs naturally as connected strand-like chains of protein enzyme molecules... amazing natural cleansing, healing, and energizing health qualities."[10] |

Some Attributes of Processed or Artificial Food Products:	Some Attributes of Pure and Wholesome Food Products:
American Processed Cheese-food	*European Raw Milk Cheese or Whole Milk Cheese*
Full of water, emulsifying agents, artificial colors, and preservatives. When heated, it easily melts, and the oil does not separate from it—again, another convenience food which our bodies cannot digest very well—there are few nutrients there for it to digest. "Cheese food" is required to contain from 50-80% natural cheese.	Made with raw, unpasteurized milk that has been raised the European way without genetically modified grain or growth hormones for the milk cows. Pasteurization destroys the enzymes by the use of chemicals, and it encourages milk intolerance. Raw milk cheese, as well as good whole milk cheese, is cured and aged for months or even years, and the ingredient list of fine imported cheese will list only "milk, rennet, and salt."
Pancake Syrup	*Pure Maple Syrup*
Made with high fructose corn syrup (see below), artificial color and flavor, preservatives, and diluted with water.	A minimally-refined, natural and nutritious sugar, rich in trace minerals. Making syrup from the concentrated sap of maple trees is a time-honored art.
High Fructose Corn Syrup	*Honey*
Contributes to similar health problems as refined sugar. Made from genetically modified corn. Corn syrup constitutes 55% of the 120 pounds of sugar per year that Americans consume; (the sugar consumption statistic was 5 pounds per year before the twentieth century.) HFCS was developed in 1967; per capita consumption was one pound in 1972 and up to ten pounds per capita by 1974.[11] Feedlot cattle that are fed and fattened on high-fructose corn develop tumors and would die before butchering time were it not for antibiotics to keep them alive. People do not fare much better on the syrup from high fructose corn. Corn syrup is in practically everything that is conventionally processed—particularly sodas and snacks.	Nature's only pre-digested food and the only natural sugar that can be eaten raw with no separating or heating. Honey contains all the nutrients that bees derive from plant pollen. Honey is replete with digestive enzymes and anti-bacterial qualities. It is relatively easy to digest, and does not raise blood sugar as much as refined white sugar does. Honey will last essentially forever in a sealed container; it is its own preservative. Honey has been discovered, perfectly edible, in Egyptian tombs—the only all-natural food that preserves itself. Processed food made with hydrogenated oil and corn syrup will last for years, appallingly, without being eaten by mold or insects, but only because man has altered it. If it's protected from insects, honey, which God wisely designed, both nourishes the body and can last forever.

Some Attributes of Processed or Artificial Food Products:	Some Attributes of Pure and Wholesome Food Products:
Flavored Ice Cream	*Natural Ice Cream*
"Synthetic from start to finish." For instance, piperonal, an artificial vanilla-like flavor, is a chemical otherwise used to kill lice. Butyraldehyde is a nut flavor otherwise used in the production of rubber cement. These are not listed in the ingredients because they are used in manufacturing.[12] Conventional ice cream is full of poor quality milk, hydrogenated oils, and corn syrup.	Some all-natural ice cream brands contain only whole milk, cream, and sugar. The oil used is often coconut oil and any flavorings are natural: peppermint oil, pure Dutch cocoa, and natural guar gum as a stabilizer. If one is going to eat ice cream, though it is usually agreed to be unhealthy, avoid the worst possible (conventional) kind! Get pure, organic ice cream for simplicity of digestion and assimilation of healthy milk and cream.
Milk Chocolate Candy	*Dark Chocolate Bar*
The first ingredient of milk chocolate is sugar, and candies are usually made with hydrogenated oils and artificial flavors. This kind of chocolate is unhealthy; any benefits of raw cocoa are outweighed by the oils, sugars, and flavors in milk chocolate. Candy bars, for the last sixty years, have been coated with cocoa and oil instead of chocolate[13]—just another way to cheapen them. Inferior-type chocolates are related to disrupted facial complexions. Quality chocolate, however, will not cause skin disruption in the same way.	Dark chocolate is high in antioxidants and is healthy except for the added sugar. Organic or natural brands usually have far more chocolate than sugar content (often from 60-80% cocoa), and are made with cocoa butter, natural vanilla extract, and other wholesome ingredients. This is the healthiest kind of chocolate and is said to have real benefits, of which conventional chocolate-flavored candies have absolutely none.

Some Attributes of Processed or Artificial Food Products:	Some Attributes of Pure and Wholesome Food Products:
Refined Sugar	*Evaporated Cane Juice Crystals*
Refined sugar has no nutritional value whatsoever. Yet these "empty calories" comprise one-fourth of caloric consumption in the Standard American Diet. Sugar contributes to bone loss and tooth decay. The B vitamins in unrefined sugar, vitamins of which refined sugar has been stripped, are necessary to help regulate blood sugar levels. Without the stabilization from B vitamins, white sugar has disastrous effects and has been called the number-one murderer of humankind and the greatest evil of industrial civilization.[14] Sugar, in one form or another, is found in practically everything processed, and, combined with other additives such as preservatives, salt, and chemical flavorings, is extremely addictive. Some commercial cereals are twenty-nine percent sugar![15] Sugar is highly addictive. Try to be disciplined not to eat it, and you will notice a craving. Replace it with healthier foods and you will slowly retrain your taste buds to like other things. From experience, I know that after trying to stay away from the sweet snacks and desserts I used to love, sugary foods are hardly even appealing anymore. Sugar will be advertised as pure if nothing else has been processed in. Well, as one author writes, "everything *has* been processed *out* of sugar but the calories."[16] It may be "pure," but it has undergone unnatural processing and is exceedingly unwholesome.	Cane juice crystals can be used in almost the same way as granulated sugar. Evaporated cane crystals have no nutrients removed, unlike typical white or brown sugar. Evaporated cane juice crystals, sucanat (dried natural cane juice), and raw turbinado crystals are all made from the evaporated juice from the whole sugar cane. Rapadura™ whole cane sugar is squeezed and dried but unrefined. Any kind of sugar is good only in moderation, but at least all of the possible nutrients in this kind will be intact. Always eats sweets with fats for better, slower absorption. While sugar is often equated with expressions of affection (candy on birthdays and chocolate on holidays), truly thoughtful love will be expressed in a way that enriches one's health rather than slowly contributing to a loved one's demise. Gifts, snacks, teatime, and receptions are all too often offerings of refined sugar. We need to stop eating so much sugar (Americans consume twenty-two pounds per capita); when we do consume sugar, we need to eat it in the most natural, nutrient-retaining form. There are many nutritious snacks that can be substituted for sugary ones: fresh fruits and vegetables, homemade naturally-sweetened cookies, yogurt, popcorn, frozen fruit juice, dried fruit, or nuts. "Once sugar is withdrawn from the diet, all foods start to taste better."[17]

Some Attributes of Processed or Artificial Food Products:	Some Attributes of Pure and Wholesome Food Products:
Aspartame	*Stevia or Agave Nectar*
Aspartame, an artificial sweetener approved by the FDA in 1981, [18] turns to poisonous formaldehyde above 86 degrees—which is within the range of body temperature. Aspartame, in independent studies, has been linked to many neurological diseases, including seizures, Alzheimer's, memory loss, and brain tumors, though the manufacturers (with money and the FDA behind them) deny these associations. It is known that aspartame contributes to weight gain because people eat more refined carbohydrates than they would otherwise.	For those people who, for immediate medical reasons, cannot eat sugar, stevia is a good alternative. It is the dried, sweet powder of the leaves of the stevia plant, is 300 times sweeter than the same amount of sugar, and is a low-carbohydrate sweetener.
As with other food products, there are claims for the verity of both sides regarding the safety of aspartame. Those who have denied the value of aspartame have proven their case by conducting many studies. I think the producers of artificial substitutes should show that it acts the same as the natural product for a long period of time before ever introducing it to the market. It should be assumed that natural things are the standard which artificial things must measure up to (which, of course, they likely never will). Fortunately, with aspartame, the truth is more well-known than it used to be. For instance, on the first page of a quick internet search, ten out of fourteen results for "aspartame" were toxicity warnings.	Agave nectar, extracted from the nectar of the cactus, is a sugar alternative that is high in fructose but is low-glycemic. It is still refined and processed, but is said to be better for dieters and diabetics than sugar is, one reason being that agave is used in smaller quantities.
Monosodium Glutamate (MSG)	*Real Food*
Monosodium glutamate is a "neurotoxic additive" used to enhance flavor in practically everything processed. It is addictive, damages the brain, and has been connected to birth defects and premenstrual syndrome, yet it is used in most Chinese restaurants and in most U.S. food manufacturing. Restaurants that make some of their food from mixes (soups, dressings, sauces, etc.) usually use products with MSG in them.	Real, natural, unprocessed food has the nutrients retained in it, not hidden by preservatives, so it has no need for artificial enhancement. Organic food in which there are more nutrients in the growing and in the processing doesn't need artificial flavor to make it palatable. MSG is banned from all certified-organic food and from all baby food.
MSG was first marketed in 1947; twenty-one years later, dizziness, headache, and chest pains were starting to be linked to MSG.	

Some Attributes of Processed or Artificial Food Products:	Some Attributes of Pure and Wholesome Food Products:
Certified USDA Hamburgers/Corn-fed Ground Beef	*Certified Organic Hamburgers/Grass-fed Ground Beef*
There are a lot of problems with the fat in conventional hamburgers, not to mention the meat. The hard layer fat (biblically unclean) has been added back in. And this fat is, to start with, unhealthy saturated fat because of being raised on grain in feedlots. If the meat is grilled, this same unhealthy fat drips onto the flames, causing carcinogens to form. We need many dark green vegetables (not just the typical iceberg lettuce) to counteract the results of grilling. Soybeans and corn are used to fatten cows in a short amount of time; it should be no surprise that the meat is fattening to humans. Soybeans and corns cause tumors in cattle. Soybeans and corn are not meant for cattle; and the cattle fed on those foods are not meant for our consumption. Feedlot-raised meat is less-expensive than ever before in history, and people eat more of it than ever before.	It is possible to get organic hamburger meat with little-to-no added fat. If raised organically, the meat will be nutritious. If it is grilled, dark green leafy vegetables need to be eaten alongside to counteract the carcinogens produced by the open flames. Organic meat may be more expensive, but taking into account that less fat will drip, and that vitamins, minerals, good fats, and rich proteins will truly nourish you, organic meat is worth its value. Unless the meat in a supermarket is certified organic or 100% grass fed, assume it came from a feedlot.

Did you know that monkeys will not eat the peels from conventionally-grown bananas, but they will eat the peels from organic bananas? Some domestic cats show great preference to organic meat versus generic meat. Animals can tell the difference between the pure versus impure foods that I give examples of in the above charts. Ants will not eat their way through white flour (preferring rather to hike around a pile of it on the ground) but they will eat right through a pile of whole wheat flour. Did you know that hamburgers from fast food restaurants and cakes packaged for long shelf life, both full of hydrogenated oils or preservatives, will not deteriorate, only dry out? Living things, whether bacteria, mold, or pests, will not assault such food-type products. We need to "Go to the ant, thou sluggard; consider her ways, and be wise: which having no guide, overseer, or ruler, provideth her meat in the summer, and gathereth her food in the harvest" (Prov. 6:6–8). We should consider the instinctive ways of God's creatures and learn from their innocent simplicity.

Here is another thought regarding animals. People often feed their animals very specific diets so that they will have optimum performance. Work horses and race horses are fed good quality hay and clover, not stubbly straw. Cattle are prescribed a combination of feed in order to mature in due time. Show animals can be fed foods that will keep their coats shiny. If this is true for animals, why not for people? After all, some groups of people, such as athletes or babies, do follow specific diets. Every person should think about whether the food he or she is eating is designed to yield optimum health and performance.

The next chart compares the two extremes of something artificial and harmful with something natural and life-giving. The chart after that compares something processed and biblically unclean with something hunted and biblically clean. Should we eat strawberry-flavored food or real strawberries? Should we eat filthy meat from a factory or pure meat from the wilderness and small farm pastures? Of course, you can acquire food flavored with real strawberries instead of the real fruit; you can acquire pasture-raised pork at a grocery store. My point is not to deny intermediate ground between the two extremes, but rather to show the differences between a type of real food and a type of adulterated food. Please note the comparisons below.

Artificial Strawberry Flavor and Color: *Benzyl-acetate, Carmine, and Red Dye No. 40*	Fresh, Real Strawberries: *Fragaria ananassa*
"A typical **artificial strawberry flavor**, like the kind found in a Burger King® strawberry milk shake, contains the following ingredients: amyl acetate, amyl butyrate, amyl valerate, anethol, anisyl formate, benzyl acetate, benzyl isobutyrate, butyric acid, cinnamyl isobutyrate, cinnamyl valerate, cognac essential oil, diacetyl, dipropyl ketone, ethyl acetate, ethyl amyl ketone, ethyl butyrate, ethyl cinnamate, ethyl heptanoate, ethyl heptylate, ethyl lactate, ethyl methylphenylglycidate, ethyl nitrate, ethyl propionate, ethyl valerate, heliotropin, hydroxyphenyl-2-butanone (10 percent solution in alcohol), a-ionone, isobutyl anthranilate, isobutyl butyrate, lemon essential oil, maltol, 4-methylacetophenone, methyl anthranilate, methyl benzoate, methyl cinnamate, methyl heptine carbonate, methyl naphthyl ketone, methyl salicylate, mint essential oil, neroli essential oil, nerolin, neryl isobutyrate, orris butter, phenethyl alcohol, rose, rum ether, g-undecalactone, vanillin, and solvent."[19] Our sense of food consists of both flavor and appearance, or color; hence, artificially flavored foods are colored red for the consumer, using one of the following: *Carmine,* which is ground-up red beetles; or, *Red No. 40,* an artificial color derived from coal-tar and petrochemicals like all artificial dyes, and a color which has replaced Red. No. 2, a dye determined to be carcinogenic after fifteen years on the market. European associations recommend that children do not consume Red No. 40. In the U.S., Red No. 40 is used even in children's medications. Artificial dyes are widely documented as contributing to hyperactivity and nervous system disorders. Red Dye No. 2 was on the market long enough for adverse side effects to be noticed and addressed, then the dye was banned. Do we think current colors and flavorings are any different? Red No. 40 is already linked to adverse side affects, but the FDA does not consider it adverse enough to be banned, if it ever is. If something is artificial, we are not meant to eat it, and its harm will therefore be felt, in some level, at some point—undeniably. Marketing on false pretenses to trusting consumers—marketing as good food what has not yet been confirmed to be harmless—is wrong. At least we can make the choice not to purchase it.	**Fresh strawberry** characteristics: High amounts of Vitamin C and the mineral manganese. Good source of iodine, omega-3 fatty acids, vitamin B6, potassium, and trace minerals. Significant rates of antioxidants which fight free-radicals—the elements that damage and alter cells. "Phytonutrients" that protect against heart disease and cancer. "Anthocyanins" that protect cell structures and prevent organ damage. Prevents macular degeneration and arthritis. Wards off toxins in blood. Cleanses skin whether taken internally or applied topically. High dietary fiber; one serving contains twelve percent of Recommended Daily Allowance for fiber. According to one list, one of eight foods linked to lower cancer rates. Most popular berry in the world. Six hundred delicious, nutritious varieties of the strawberry have been classified. We are instinctively attracted to brightly colored foods as these contain the most nutrients, especially vitamins. Strawberries meet these criteria excellently! Real strawberries consist completely of goodness that God designed to nourish us. Eating a serving of fresh strawberries provides hydration, fiber, vitamins, and minerals. The world's favorite berry has been cultivated for millennia to the great delight of all who have eaten it. The bright color and appealing texture of strawberries invites us to partake pleasurably and beneficially of its nutrients. God designed fruit to be attractive; and we are amply rewarded with contributions to our health when we consume it.

Along the interstate, my family has driven past feedlots for hogs and cattle, and we have flown above feedlots in small-engine planes. The characteristic stench of manure is repulsive and overwhelming, and there is not a blade of grass in sight; we do all we can to get far away from such places. Few things smell worse on a hot July day.

In the mountains, my family has often hiked in the habitat of deer and elk. The fragrance from the pine trees, grasses, streams, and wildflowers is so inviting and refreshing that we do all we can to enjoy the outdoors as often as possible. When we have shot deer for our consumption, we are greeted with the welcome aroma of fresh game. Few things smell better on a crisp October day.

Between factory pork and wild deer, I wonder which animals are happier? I ask this question not out of concern for so-called animal rights, but because the Bible speaks of the animals, praising Him from the environment that is their habitat, and says that "a righteous man regardeth the life of his beast" (Prov. 12:10). Animals do not consciously praise God as far as we know, but He is evidently glorified by their natural existence. I wonder if our initial impression of a food or its source has anything to do with whether we should be eating it. I believe that it does, and so contends the following quotation. Action must begin to meet intuition.

The bottom line is this: a farm friendly food system is both aromatically and aesthetically pleasing. Anything else is not a good food system, period...Intuitively we understand all of this and yet our culture continues to defend a food system that is neither pretty nor aromatically pleasing.[20]

Factory-farmed Pork: *Sus scrofa domesticus*	Wild Venison (Deer): *Odocoileus virginianus*
Characteristics of factory-produced **pork**:	Characteristics of **venison** gleaned from the wild:
Source of unhealthy saturated fat (due to the content of their feed.)	Excellent, healthy source of protein.
The "effect of pork consumption on blood chemistry" is shown in the observation of "serious changes for several hours after pork is consumed"—even with organic pork. "In the laboratory, pork is one of the best mediums for feeding the growth of cancer cells."[21]	Rich in minerals, especially iron. The iron in venison is more easily absorbed than that in beef. Rich in B vitamins, which are vitamins often lacking in carbohydrate-laden diets.
"Over seventy percent of pork producers use a carcinogenic drug called sulfamethazine as a growth stimulant and to control rampant diseases."[22]	Good source of healthy, natural saturated fats (due to the nature of their diet). Deer are lean, and their saturated fats are some of the best known, since deer have fed on a diet of grasses.
Pigs are housed in Confined Animal Feeding Operations, which are "breeding grounds for disease"[23] and which can handle 80,000 sows a year, fattening them in only five and a half months.[24]	One source believes venison to be healthier than turkey—and turkey is widely claimed to be a "super-food."
Pigs are "kept alive until the moment of slaughter" by supporting their overburdened, sickly bodies until the point at which they are both large enough to slaughter yet too weak to live on their own.	Native people groups relying on hunting and gathering would harvest older male animals—the ones with the most fat—as this meat supplied much of the fat in their diet if they didn't have access to oils.
Feedlot animals are raised on food which, in large amounts, is toxic to their organs; they are treated with steroids to fatten quickly; and they are given antibiotics to keep them alive despite filthy conditions.	Wild game is not only very nutritious; hunting it is akin to the same process that has been followed for millennia—unlike feedlots and factories that have sprung up in the last sixty years.
I know some people are so emotionally connected with the taste of pork that they think they could scarcely do without it. However, the Christian way is to consult what is wise and truthful instead of being led by our feelings and emotions.	I know some people are queasy at the thought of hunting. If so, they are too removed from the origins of food. Some people would rather open a package without thinking about where food comes from. People in the Bible hunted, and hunting is one of the best ways to know your food supply. God has given man the ability to raise domesticated animals, but He has provided animals in the wilderness for our sustenance as well. Hunting is an area of taking dominion, of providing for one's family, and of being economical in the acquisition of healthy meat.
Pork is filthy, filthy, filthy all the way from the food hogs eat, to the way it is digested, to the conditions of factories, to the effects that pork has on the human body.	
Pork originating from feedlots has gone through so many stages that the average consumer has no idea of the processes used. In fact, if everyone knew how much animals were confined, how their systems were taxed by unnatural substances, and how they are slaughtered in massive numbers, people who typically don't like hunting might start to think that hunting is far more humane.	Venison that has been hunted in the wild is only two steps away from the dining room table. Venison is one of the most local, fresh products that can be acquired.
	Deer that live all of their lives on the open range of their habitat right up until the moment of a hunter's harvest have lived much better than feedlot pigs.
The hogs are raised to exactly specified standards so that they are as identical in age and size as possible and more easily move through the slaughter process.	The differences in species and habits of deer, as well as their varying sizes and their unique antlers, display the diversity that God created.

Not only are the ingredients of conventional versus organic food vastly different, as seen above, but the packaging on foods can be worlds apart. Conventional food is advertised largely on the basis of how exciting it is and why it will make you happy, make you feel good, make your life easier, help you to have fun, or whatever other gimmicks can be given. Given the awful, actual processes and hidden, filler ingredients in much processed food, it should be no surprise that giant food companies lobby Congress for allowance to disclose as little as possible of the truth about their products. It is lawful, for instance, to use dangerous MSG under the listing of "natural flavors."

Packaging claims are sometimes made based on the traditional value of foods: that milk and beef are good for you (they are, only in their natural, unchanged forms); that "Grandma's kitchen" or "home-cooking" are the healthiest choices (this is true, but modern factories are light-years removed); that cold cereal is a good source of fiber (it may have a little fiber, but not compared to the amount of fiber in home-cooked whole grain oatmeal). Packages of conventionally-produced food tend to focus on how much (size, value, etc.) you are getting for your money; how ready it is to use (scoop, spread, sprinkle, etc.); and how it appears (the shape of the product, the colorful packaging, etc.) to the consumer. One observation is that large food corporations (applicable to either manufacturers or restaurants) are mostly in the entertainment business.[25]

A number of packaged foods, that I have noticed lately, advertise a certain *real* ingredient, such as soup mix made with *real* onions, or popcorn made with *real* butter. How far we have come, shamefully, when food has to be marketed as "real" to distinguish it from the alternative!

If consumers buy foods that excite or instantly gratify themselves, then producers will manufacture foods to impress consumers. The theme of the conventional American food industry is to produce ever bigger, ever cheaper, and ever faster. A better quality or the best quality is never considered.[26] A mediocre quality is seemingly acceptable as long as the first purposes—income and gratification—are met. To quote Joel Salatin again, regarding the commercial propensity to generate the biggest cows, biggest ears of corn, biggest apples, and biggest cans of soda—"We worship growth as if it is the noblest goal in the world."[27] Are growth of weight or growth of cancer noble goals, he asks? Unqualified growth is not inherently best, yet Americans have been taught to equate value with volume—in everything from cereal boxes to government programs.

On the contrary, packages of pure, organic and natural foods tell a story about the people producing the food, the farm it is grown on, the reason for growing it, and the health advantages of the product. These companies have great stories to tell because they believe that achieving purity and quality is more fundamental than their bottom line, and they pursue this achievement regardless of the most popular methods used today.

Companies in the conventional food industry do not tell, nor would they want to tell, their true stories. Their stories would be tales of polluting the earth and air, of genetically modifying plants, of treating animals like machines, of endangering human health, and of caring little for God's creation.

Organic companies want to sell their product and make a profit, of course, and they do their marketing with this in mind. However, they market by telling the truth about their products—products they can rightfully be proud of, having produced them by considering consumers' health and the earth before their financial statements. Common to most packages of organic or purposefully natural food is the candor to tell where ingredients come from, as well as a sense of history in telling when, where, and by whom the products are made. Organic foods are developed by dairymen who love their animals, bakers who love their craft, and gardeners who love their soil.

From Organic or Natural Food Packaging:
From *Garden Time® Organic Fettuccine*: "Located hundreds of miles from any major city so our wheat is not exposed to urban chemicals and pollutants..."; "Generations of Old World Italian craftsmanship..."
From *Partners® Olive Oil and Herb Crackers*: "Using all natural ingredients while supporting the sustainability of our environment..."
From *Native Forest® Unsweetened Organic Coconut Milk*: "Devoted farmers have achieved organic certification of their traditional coconut crop..."; "An oil-rich extract that is mixed with only filtered water and a tiny amount (less than 1%) of guar gum..."
From *Organic Valley® Family of Farms Whole Milk*: "Award-winning taste from nature..."; "Shortening the distance from farm to plate..."; "High standards for animal well-being..."
From *Pacific Natural Foods® Organic Vegetable Broth*: "Our partner farms and suppliers guarantee quality and safety..."; "We know the history and origin of every ingredient..."
From *R.W. Knudsen Family™ Organic Grapefruit Juice from Concentrate*: "Commitment began with a desire to make wholesome juices of the best possible quality for his own family..."
From *Kashi Organic Promise® Island Vanilla® Organic Whole Wheat Biscuits*: "They have been handled with care from farm to market..."; "You help support the health of farmers, farm workers, livestock, and the environment."
From *Chef Bruce Aidells® Chicken and Apple Smoked Chicken Sausage*: "Zero grams trans-fat; no gluten; no MSG..."; "Chicken that has been raised without antibiotics or growth hormones..."
From *Oakdell Egg Farms® Fresh Eggs*: "10 times more vitamin E compared to a regular egg"; "Fed a vegetarian diet containing flaxseed. No hormones, antibiotics, or animal by-products..."

Following are four charts to present some basic options for purchasing or making bread and cookies and for purchasing or growing beef and tomatoes. Some of this information was discussed in my chapter on using our dollars to promote the principles we believe in; however, these charts should provide a useful, more detailed comparison in relation to some of the nutrition facts we have been considering in this chapter.

Possible Bread Choices from Worst to Best
Commercial White Bread: Ingredients of most of the loaves of bread found in a grocery store contain enriched white flour, several kinds of processed sweeteners including corn syrup, hydrogenated oils, dough conditioners and preservatives, natural and artificial flavors, and fewer grams of fiber than of sugar.
Organic Wheat Bread: A better choice is all-natural (or organic) whole grain, even gluten-free, bread made with whole grain flours, natural sweeteners such as honey or molasses, healthy oils, and sea salt. Whole grain bread is high in fiber. If you buy bread without preservatives, it will need to be fairly local to taste fresh and remain unspoiled for a few days.
Homemade Bread: One of the best choices is to make fresh homemade bread with organic and natural ingredients. My family has made the majority of our bread, especially our sandwich bread, for ten years. The wheat that we grind is grown by a local company, is non-genetically modified, and has no traceable levels of pesticides. Our raw honey comes from our own beehives or a local beekeeper, and the extra-virgin olive oil we use is imported from Italy.
Sprouted Grain Bread: Some health experts advocate that, in bread making, grain should be sprouted or flour should be soaked ahead of time, for easier digestion and assimilation of nutrients. Numerous companies sell sprouted whole grain bread in supermarkets. Soaking, for partial breakdown and fermentation of flour, can be achieved by making bread with sourdough, buttermilk, or yogurt.

Possible Cookie Choices from Worst to Best
Conventional Store-bought Cookies: Typical packaged chocolate cookies contain white flour, refined sugars, bad fats, artificial flavors, sweetened additive-laden chocolate, and preservatives, and are neither fresh nor local.
Specialty Cookies: Gourmet-type store-bought cookies usually have natural and better quality (real) ingredients, although refined. Organic store-bought cookies, likewise, have natural ingredients: most notably organic flour, natural sweeteners, healthy oils, and if there is chocolate, organic chocolate.

Homemade Cookies: Homemade cookies can be made with conventional ingredients, such as white flour and shortening, and would be hardly any healthier than typical packaged cookies except that they would be fresher and have no need of preservatives. Making cookies at home, however, is a great and economical opportunity to use the same natural ingredients that you should use in other baking, including whole, fiber-rich grains and unrefined sweeteners. If you make things yourself, you can govern a healthy outcome by cutting back on sugar and adding more fiber in the form of wheat germ or flaxseed.

Alternative Options: Some nutritionists advocate eating no commercially-made or unsoaked grain products—of which cookies, crackers, and cakes are the prime culprits. These products are high in sugar and flour: refined carbohydrates. If a person gets enough good fats and good proteins in their diet, cravings for sugar will decrease and their small desire for sweets can easily be satisfied with a few pieces of dried fruit or a square of barely-sweetened dark chocolate. Many recipes are available for cookies and bars made with mostly fruit and nuts, which can be much healthier than the typical flour-sugar-oil composition.

Various Ways of Purchasing Meat, from Worst to Best

Conventionally-grown Meat: Buy meat from a grocery store where it has been shipped across the nation, where the meat has gone through countless hands, where you have no personal contact with or knowledge about the process, where you can be sure the meat has been raised in the filthiest confined conditions and loaded with nitrates, and where your money goes to support more of the same.

Organic Meat: Buy meat from an organic regional company that discloses exactly how the meat is produced and certifies it as such, tells you what they believe in and why, and covets your purchase as support for their good and principled efforts.

Local Grass-fed Meat: Buy meat locally from a grower whom you can meet, who has an interest in the community and his customers' health, whose farm you can see for yourself, whose food is not only nutritious, but local and fresh, and whose family you support with your purchase. Joel Salatin has said, "The 'get-big' mentality has fostered corner-cutting and inappropriate procedures that would never have been done under the careful scrutiny—relationship—of both producer and consumer."[28] Having met his customers, a grower feels more responsible. Where a friendly relationship exists, customers are more likely to pay a higher price for the product, since part of what you pay for is the experience received and the trust shared.

Homegrown Meat: Raise domestic animals yourself or hunt game animals (elk, venison, and game birds). From personally raising meat, you will know exactly what is put into it and will have your own good quality meat for the lowest possible cost. This method is the way to have the most personal involvement with the acquisition of food. There is nothing spiritual about this process; it is simply the most economical and most healthful.

Various Ways to Purchase Tomatoes, from Worst to Best
Conventional produce: Conventional tomatoes have low-nutrients (evidenced by their pale color) and residual pesticides, are often unripe when picked, and are shipped across the nation.
Organic produce: Organic, regionally grown tomatoes are free of pesticide residue and are often more brightly colored, and therefore more nutrient-rich, than their counterparts, but are usually shipped considerable distances.
Local produce: Farmers' Markets or Community Supported Agriculture or cooperatives are good places to find fresh produce locally grown and often organic, whether or not it is certified.
Homegrown produce: A personal garden is the best way to ensure the purity of your vegetables and control the whole environment from planting to harvesting. This method is again the most economical, especially when you can preserve the abundance for winter.

The following chart addresses a different theme from the above comparisons. The merits and detriments of fats and oils have been addressed numerous times, as have the place that oils have in the standard American diet, the cuisine of the Mediterranean, and on tropical islands. Below, the consumption of fats and oils in those three regions are listed side by side, as are the health conditions evident from the typical countries on these diets.

With the below chart, I conclude this chapter. In the next chapter, even more practical tips for shopping and selecting will be presented.

Mediterranean Coast: Oil Consumption	Polynesian Islands: Oil Consumption	United States: Oil Consumption
Diet comprised of 40% fat.	Diet comprised of 40% fat.	Diet comprised of 40% fat.
Types of oils: monounsaturated olive oil, nuts and nut oils, avocadoes, wild-caught fish, raw or whole milk cheeses. (Mostly monounsaturated fat.)	Types of oils: healthy saturated coconut oil and coconuts, wild-caught fish, oils from other nuts and plants. (Mostly saturated fat.)	Types of oils: polyunsaturated, hydrogenated vegetable oils from corn, soy, canola, and cottonseed; unhealthy saturated fat from grain-fed beef and pork. (Mostly trans-fats.)
Fats and oils are used in cooking, sautéing, salads, salad dressings, and on their own (in the case of cheese, meat, and fish).	Fats and oils are found in raw or simply-prepared foods; coconut is a mainstay of the diet and is used in a wide variety of ways.	High proportion of fat coming from saturated fat in conventional red meat. Hydrogenated oils are used in margarine spreads, bakery items, and nearly all processed foods.

Mediterranean Coast: Oil Consumption	Polynesian Islands: Oil Consumption	United States: Oil Consumption
High Omega-3 content. Ratio of Omega-6 and Omega-3 fatty acids is roughly 1:1, the delicate balance which the body needs.	High Omega-3 content. Ratio of Omega-6 and Omega-3 fatty acids is roughly 1:1, the delicate balance which the body needs.	Low Omega-3 content. High Omega-6 content. Ratio of Omega-6 and Omega-3 fatty acids is from 10:1 to 20:1, extremely out of balance and paving the pathway to disease.
Principle: Good fats prevent disease.	Principle: Good fats prevent disease.	Principle: Bad fats cause disease.
Low rates of cardiovascular disease and cancer; less body fat and longer life span than those on typical Western diet. Oils from the purest sources provide protection from the sunshine and an outdoor lifestyle.	Low rates of disease; excellent immunity and physical stamina; most ideal body structure that has been observed. Antiviral qualities of coconut are perfect for protection in tropical environments.	Cardiovascular disease number one killer, followed by cancer and other degenerative diseases. Compromised mental and physical function due to major fat imbalance makes people susceptible to many ailments.

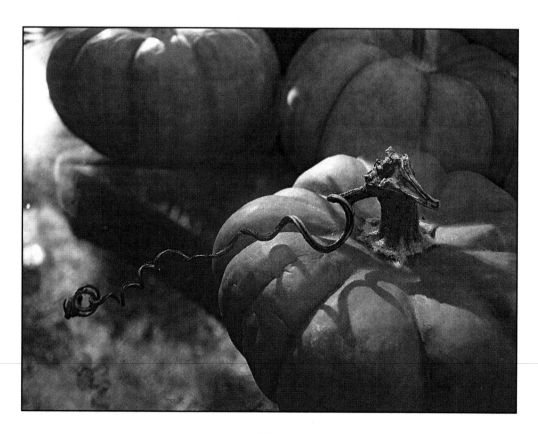

Chapter Twenty-two

Health-Conscious Shopping

"Whatever the father of illness, the mother is the wrong food."[1]
—Chinese Proverb

AS YOU SEEK to understand a healthy diet—consisting of healthful foods—you will notice that just about every single ingredient will require attention, from salt to strawberries to salmon. If you desire to make a few lifestyle changes, start thinking about every single product in your cupboard, refrigerator, and freezer (as well as laundry and vanity cabinets, for that matter). Gradually, start purging every item you have and seek to replace it. Pay attention to and replace your previously habitual purchases with thoughtful, deliberate purchases. Nothing is neutral; everything will take analysis and a decision.

In our family, we buy basically nothing from generic brands except for a few single-ingredient foods—and anymore, hardly at all. Name-brand conglomerates manufacture things in the unpleasant ways discussed in past chapters. How accustomed we get to particular brands is surprising—at other people's homes I am sometimes surprised at the brands of their food because we have not used them in years. On the other hand, the organic brands we customarily use probably look unusual to someone not used to them.

Think of grocery shopping as a treasure hunt to find gems of purity, health, and goodness. Do not take things at face value. Search deeper—read the labels and apply all of the things you have learned about food. When I was quite young, I once asked my mom why the ingredients were printed on the box—and why anyone cared. Well, now I definitely know! Reading labels does involve time, but consider this idea: you are informing and educating yourself while also protecting yourself from injurious ingredients. For the next part of this chapter, a sample shopping list is provided. While far from exhaustive, the list should help to solidify and give shape to some of the principles we have dealt with earlier.

In *A Field Guide to Buying Organic*, the authors encourage knowing the stories and the culture associated with food. Simply start to think more about your shopping, and you'll suddenly become a shaper of a better culture rather than a buyer at the mercy of the existing culture.

> Because we Americans have been blessed with a plentiful and inexpensive food supply, we don't often take the time to think about the impact of our food purchases. We make decisions on every trip to the grocery store, but beyond the shelf and behind the labels, there's a story to tell. How our food is produced directly affects the life and health of our culture. It's about you, your family, your community, all of us: shuffling through the aisles, holding options to the light, comparing apples with apples.[2]

A Suggested Basic Shopping List:

Meats: Pasture-raised biblically-clean meats and poultry and wild-caught ocean fish (from filets, to ground meat, to sausage, to lunch meat, as long as it is additive-free). Beef, wild game, lamb, turkey, chicken, salmon, and more. It should be understood that biblically-unclean animals *are* by nature scavengers or filters and are conventionally raised in the worst conditions of all; so, if eaten, organic versions are imperative.

Dairy: Organic milk (raw if possible) from free-range cows. Organic cream and buttermilk. Organic sour cream and yogurt or natural sour cream and yogurt with no added sugars or preservatives. Hormone-free cow's milk cheeses, whether European-produced or domestically-produced but specified as such; (imported raw or whole milk cheeses can be less expensive than domestic organic cheeses.) Sheep's milk and goat's milk cheeses. Free-range eggs high in omega-3 fatty acids.

Fats: Butter from free-range cattle, extra-virgin olive oil, and extra-virgin coconut oil, all high in omega-3s. Cod liver oil (as a supplement, not for cooking). Organic cold-pressed peanut, safflower, and sunflower oils are technically stable and are safe vegetable oils for human consumption, but are high in omega-6 fatty acids and should be used in moderation.

Grains: Non-genetically modified whole grains for home-grinding or for hot cereal, or non-genetically modified whole grain flours for baking and cooking (wheat, cracked wheat, barley, millet, oats, corn, brown rice, polenta, couscous, and more). Whole grain loaves of bread and other bread products: sourdough, soaked, or sprouted is thought to be optimum. Pastas, bagels, chips, crackers, and cold cereals should be minimally used—only buy these whole grain and all-natural, even organic.

Legumes, nuts, and seeds: Beans, nuts, and seeds: beans are best soaked and cooked at home (and frozen for future use) rather than canned. Nuts and seeds, which grow with shells, are not a necessary item to buy organic, but are more easily digested if they have been soaked and dried first. Buy nuts whole; they can go rancid after they've been chopped.

Produce: Fresh fruits and vegetables should be bought organic if possible. The kinds of produce that are less important to buy organic tend to have thicker skins, are less susceptible to insects, and therefore less in need of or susceptible to pesticides: broccoli, eggplant, cabbage, asparagus, peas, onions, sweet potatoes, watermelon, avocadoes, bananas, pineapple, mangoes, and kiwis. Those kinds of produce with thinner skins, especially fruit, are soaked with pesticides and are best if bought organic to lessen pesticide residue: apples, pears, peaches, strawberries, raspberries, cherries, grapes, bell peppers, green beans, celery, cucumbers, tomatoes, spinach, lettuce, potatoes, and carrots.
With any produce, it is advantageous to use an organic produce wash (often citrus- or coconut-based) to remove the surface sprays, waxes, or bacteria. Using produce wash on all produce, both organic and conventional, is a wise step beyond the mere, and often forgotten, rinsing with water.
Corn and soybeans are usually heavily sprayed and genetically modified so are best to buy organic (as well as organic versions of products containing any corn or soybean derivatives). Fresh or frozen produce retains more nutrients than canned versions. If bought, buy canned fruit without added sugar and canned vegetables without added salt. It may be very hard to find nice-looking organic fruit and vegetables out of season (chemical sprays keep conventional produce looking nice all year long), so buy naturally-grown produce in bulk from regional growers at the time of harvest and preserve the excess for the rest of the year.
All *organic* food is non-genetically modified, but if you buy conventionally-grown produce, try to get it non-GMO. A Price Look-Up (PLU) code (on the sticker) with five numbers beginning with the number 9 is organic. A PLU code with five numbers beginning with the number 8 is genetically modified. A PLU code with four numbers beginning with the number 4 is conventionally-grown with the use of pesticides and herbicides. However, dairy products, meats, oils, and whole grain products are viewed to be the best

foods to spend your allotted "organic/natural dollars" on than on produce, if you cannot afford to buy everything organic. It should be noted that genetically modified foods used in *products* are *not* revealed—GMOs are only revealed on the stickers of fresh produce.

Sugars: Honey, maple syrup, date sugar, molasses, stevia, and agave nectar. Evaporated cane juice crystals, sucanat (sugar cane natural) or raw turbinado sugar—the least refined cane sugars.

Condiments: Raw apple cider vinegar, Balsamic vinegar, red wine vinegar, Celtic sea salt, pure dried herbs and spices, naturally-fermented soy sauce, organic ketchup and mustard, olive oil or safflower mayonnaise (not canola, soybean or vegetable oil mayonnaise.) It is best to make your own sauces, syrups, and dressings with wholesome ingredients, but if you buy these things, look for all-natural or organic varieties that contain good or zero sugars as well as good oils (for instance, olive oil and honey, not canola oil and corn syrup).

Beverages: Water (preferably from a well or spring or filtered—not chemically treated in any way); herbal and decaffeinated teas; fresh vegetable and fruit juices. Coffee, sodas, and alcohol should be used only occasionally and in moderation (if at all) and should all be bought in organic versions.

Naturally-fermented (soured, with good bacteria) foods and drinks are highly recommended in *Nourishing Traditions* and other whole food cookbooks as a way to eat milk, vegetables, condiments, and beverages.

Super-foods: The following foods have particularly high concentrations of healthful phytonutrients and should be incorporated into meals whenever possible.

- Apples
- Avocadoes
- Bananas
- Beans & lentils
- Beets
- Blackberries
- Blueberries
- Broccoli
- Cabbage

- Cherries
- Chocolate, dark, raw
- Coconut oil
- Cod liver oil
- Cranberries
- Flaxseed
- Ginger
- Green tea
- Kale

- Nuts & seeds
- Oatmeal
- Oranges
- Quinoa
- Pomegranate
- Pumpkin
- Raspberries
- Red onions
- Salmon

- Spinach
- Spirulina
- Strawberries
- Tomatoes
- Turkey
- Walnuts
- Wheat germ
- Yogurt

Prepared foods and meals: If you buy anything ready-made at the store, use discernment in the following way. Is the prepared product or mix *made with* the foods and ingredients listed above? Many natural or organic, albeit somewhat processed, products are available, from cake mixes to salad dressings to rice pilaf mixes. Buy only those products that are comprised of wholesome, pure, and real foods, and that will be a step in the right direction. Choosing organic foods will eliminate preservatives and other artificial ingredients—worse culprits than processed ingredients. Better yet, make your own mixes at home or cook the food from scratch.

Learn to distinguish, as much as you can, between "somewhat healthy" and "very unhealthy" foods. If you need to buy conventional canned soup, buy a vegetable-based one rather than a cream-based one; it will have much fewer and much simpler ingredients. If you need to buy a snack at a generic convenience store, get plain pretzels and an unsweetened iced tea rather than artificial-cheese-flavored puffs and a bottle of corn-syrupy soda.

Restaurants, traveling, visiting, and holidays: Distinguishing between foods leads to some thoughts regarding traveling. Understandably, eating properly while traveling is difficult, merely by virtue of the limited options in any one place or time. Fortunately, while homemade food is always the best choice, there are more and more whole-food and organic restaurants opening all over. Health food stores often have excellent delis and since they aren't full-service, the prices are reasonable and you can be satisfied about what you have eaten. Again, always compare options and choose the healthiest option possible. If you have a choice between Arby's® and McDonald's®, it is preferable to go where you can get a roast beef sandwich rather than a deep-fat-fried hamburger. If you have a choice between Subway® and a Chinese buffet, go where you can get a fresh sandwich rather than sweet-and-sour-chicken laced with red dye and MSG. If you go to Subway®, choose turkey rather than beef (turkey has fewer nitrates) and choose their vinegar-based dressings rather than dairy-based dressing. If you end up needing to patronize the Chinese restaurant, choose some stir-fried beef and vegetables rather than deep-fried chicken with red sweet-and-sour sauce. Do you see the increments of choices that can be made?

Generally, at restaurants with a variety of choices, I will select a vegetable dish or salad rather than a predominately-meat entrée. I can get pasture-fed meat at home; I would rather avoid conventional meats and have a hearty salad instead. (*The Maker's Diet* book recommends, however, that ordering meat at restaurants is preferable to ordering food containing refined white flour, such as pasta or pizza.) For breakfasts, order wheat toast and ask for butter; make sure the cook doesn't slather it with margarine. Ask for an omelet made with turkey or steak rather than getting pork sausage on the side. Airports are another story. Still, one can get a green salad, a taco with beans and rice, or a yogurt smoothie, and eat fairly simply.

One idea we have tried to implement is to take our own food along, in a cooler, for the first several meals of a driving trip. After that, we purchase hearty bread, cheese, yogurt, and bananas from a grocery store for further breakfasts and lunches. When you do need to choose a restaurant, keep in mind that the less expensive restaurants, and some chains or franchises, generally use mixes for a lot of dishes: pancakes, soups, dressings, puddings, etc. Mixes are notorious for containing hydrogenated oils, preservatives, MSG, and other additives. Restaurants where the food is made "from scratch," and restaurants which pride themselves on gourmet cuisine, will generally be quite a bit healthier. Basically, the most sensible advice I can give is to make an effort to choose the best option of any given selection: the healthiest restaurant in the vicinity, then the healthiest option on the menu, then the healthiest toppings or side dishes.

Similar principles apply to picnics or potlucks or even people's homes. At a buffet table, serve yourself more from the dishes that look the most healthful. This isn't a time to throw out all the rules; it's a time to exercise your knowledge and your discipline! Learn to eat the simplest food; a green salad with a choice of dressings will be more nutritious than a potato salad smothered in soybean-oil mayonnaise. A wedge of homemade peach or cherry pie will be more nutritious than an instant-pudding dessert topped with hydrogenated non-dairy whipped topping. If you are at someone's home, you may make small choices even while being served. Eat that smaller slice of pork roast and take more broccoli instead. Ask for your pound cake to be served without the whipped topping, your water to be served without ice, or your toast to be served without margarine or jelly.

As mentioned before, it is right and good to accept hospitality without becoming worrisome. Having a hospitable spirit includes not only having people into our own homes, but being content and gracious guests in the homes of those who don't cook as we might cook. A full ten percent of our health, it is believed, comes from enjoying our food—and, I would add, having an attitude of praise to God for it. Besides, if a person is healthy to start with, occasionally eating unhealthy foods will not be too detrimental. Some believe that a healthy person can handle twenty percent less-than-desirable food if we eat truly wholesome food eighty percent of the time.

Holidays need not be a time of throwing out healthful guidelines, either. In fact, it is an exciting challenge to create healthy versions of traditional foods, to make healthy snacks to please and nourish guests, and to prepare healthy desserts so you don't feel guilty eating them. In fact, some holiday meals naturally burst with superfoods as long as they are not counteracted by inadvisable foods. Free-range turkey, sweet potatoes, pumpkin, cranberries, broccoli, and other green vegetables are all wonderful foods if they are allowed to shine without being overwhelmed by refined sugar, margarine, or other rich and fattening embellishments. The next time a holiday approaches, consider it your mission to showcase the superfoods and to enhance them with wholesome seasonings. Avoid ladening the table with heavy starch and dairy in the form of buttered bread, stuffing, creamy potatoes, *and* corn pudding. Pies can be made with raw honey or maple syrup, without sugar or corn syrup.

Typical American holidays celebrate the good things that God has given us—the risen Savior on Resurrection Day, national liberty at Independence Day, a godly heritage on Thanksgiving Day, and the incarnated Son of God on Christmas Day. These ought not to be times of levity and disregard for wise principles of food and drink. Special occasions are perfect opportunities to tangibly put into practice the best things we believe about God's transformation of our lives and about the delicate freedom that is our American heritage. Our celebration can extend to the very morsels we eat, not stopping in the vague realm of happy sentiments.

Christ came to earth to transform every aspect of our lives. Colonial soldiers fought to maintain our freedom to live in liberty. May we not be ungrateful for either of these great, though far unequal, accomplishments. We are called to exercise Christian self-control, yet overindulging at special meals is thought to be normal and predictable. Our forefathers fought for limited government, yet food purchasing decisions often support the industries subsidized by the growing federal bureaucracy. Holidays are understandably a cause for celebration and for the enjoyment of special foods, but holidays need not be an excuse for unfettered eating. Holidays are a time to most carefully apply principles and standards for healthful foods, for the benefit of all that are gathered together, and out of gratitude to God.

On another note, many nutritionists suggest taking digestive enzyme tablets with meals, especially when visiting or traveling—times when the food is different from what you are (hopefully) used to. Digestive enzymes can aid in the absorption of the good nutrients in lesser-quality food and help food move through your system, rather than letting bad oils, sticky white flour, and fatty meat clog your body. These supplement tablets can be found at health food stores and are highly recommended for taking with meals away from home.

Care of food purchased: If you have spent money on good quality food and ingredients, you will want to take good care of them. Organic produce doesn't last as long as conventional produce because it hasn't been sprayed with growth inhibitors or waxes. Bread products made without preservatives will mold much sooner than generic breads. Fried foods such as potato chips or doughnuts don't rot because the frying oil that permeates the food has been so radically altered. Basically, the more processing a food has undergone, the less it will rot. Some foods are so processed that they never decay. *Real food rots*, as many nutritionists have stated. Therefore, when you buy real food you need to eat it or preserve it (freeze, dry, can, etc.) before it rots! The fresher it is, the more nutrients it retains anyway.

With any type of food preparation, food safety for the prevention of food-borne diseases is very important. Many people are not aware of the food storage and surface cleanliness guidelines that have been established for the abidance of restaurants and food service institutions. Local health departments have codes which serve as the standard for licensing and inspections. While homes are obviously not required to follow these standards, the standards reflect principles of health and safety and are helpful to know.

The major arena for the growth of bacteria, parasites, and viruses is "potentially hazardous foods." This category includes foods containing moisture or protein—mainly meat or milk products, sliced fruit, and any prepared dishes. The "danger zone" for these foods is between 41 degrees and 140 degrees Fahrenheit. Potentially-hazardous foods must be kept *colder than 41 degrees or hotter than 140 degrees* to be safe—which means to inhibit the growth of bacteria, parasites, and viruses. In our local Montana county, the regulations require that potentially hazardous food must be discarded if it has been in the danger zone for a total of *four hours* (the sum of all periods of time being served, stored, or transported). The warmer the air is, or the longer food sits in cooler air, the more bacteria will grow. For those instances, some research has indicated that even *one to two hours* sitting outside of a refrigerator or oven is long enough to spoil a potentially hazardous food. These timeframes are wise to keep in mind while preparing, serving, and putting away food before and after meals.

In the refrigerator, raw meats are not to be kept for more than four days. Opened containers of dairy products, and any prepared foods (salads, casseroles, sauces, puddings, cooked meat, cooked vegetables, etc.), are to be used within seven days. The seven-day rule does not apply to condiments, which usually have a high proportion of vinegar, sugar, or salt as preservatives. Since I always used to wonder if something was expired in the fridge or on the counter, I was pleased to learn these guidelines and hope they will be helpful to you, too.

Chapter Twenty-three

Actions Beyond Food

"The doctor of the future will give no medicine, but will interest his patients in the care of the human frame, in diet and the cause and prevention of disease."[1]
—Thomas Edison

WHILE PEOPLE WILL develop differing convictions about what contributes to health, it is important for Christians to consider a standard for health and to seek God's ways, not those of the medical industry. Christians should search for wise and proper information and approach life the best way—the healthy way.

Throughout our lives, our bodies withstand the accumulation of bad input and injuries. Knowing that damage will transpire, a prudent action is to take preventative care and dietary measures. As any tool or machine needs cleansing and repair to keep it operating at full efficiency, the human body likewise needs cleansing and care. A diet that fortifies our bodily systems is paramount in such care. Health care that fortifies is similarly advantageous.

Up until now, we have mostly surveyed the issue of health-giving diets—a vital subject, since eating concerns every living person on earth. Another key subject related to health is proper, but voluntary, professional care—such as chiropractic or dental. Meals have a necessary consistency for the prevention of hunger, but many natural health practitioners would likewise suggest consistent treatment for the prevention of disease.

If the body malfunctions, disease is bred. What, then, leads to malfunction? A poor diet and injuries that have incorrectly healed can lead to malfunction. By the time *disease* manifests itself, the body has been malfunctioning for many years. The conventional medical establishment exists to treat full-fledged disease—seldom prevention—and tends to cover symptoms rather than alleviate and remove symptoms. *Prevention* connotes working the right way from the beginning, a method completely foreign to most medical practice. Prevention is akin to the biblical principles of laying a good foundation, and of working from the inside to the outward and then upward.

Modern medicine does fill a useful place for confronting bodily crises and stepping in aggressively, for instance, to restore failed organs or provide life support. Administering medications for years on end, however, is no answer for simpler maladies that proper diet and/or chiropractic care has been known to correct in weeks or months. There are countless stories written by people who, after being told by their allopathic doctor to go home and live with their malady (or die with it as the case may be), turned to a raw food diet, a chiropractor, or to other natural health practitioners for answers and ultimately healing. Drugs attack the body and try to make it react differently to problems for which the body was manifesting a natural reaction. Sometimes, the abrupt power of drugs is quite necessary to sustain life in men, women, or children with serious chronic conditions; in this way, science has truly reached marvelous heights. Most of the time, though, a better approach is to use natural treatments which come alongside of and correct the body calmly, preventing the body from manifesting adverse reactions.

Chiropractic care, to explain further, is a field of health care which helps the body to function optimally. In the words of one chiropractic doctor, "A doctor of chiropractic is uniquely trained to locate and help correct nerve system interference which promotes the body's natural healing ability."[2] Chiropractors believe that the body has innate intelligence to heal itself when allowed to function properly. That function begins with the nervous system—one of the earliest systems formed in babies in the womb and a system which, if properly aligned, capably commands every aspect of our bodies. Since every individual has a unique composition and unique combination of needs, helping the body to return to its optimal and foundational condition is understood to be the best way to allow the body to heal and care for itself unhindered.

While a good diet is fundamental to strengthening the body, other natural, non-invasive means can be advantageous for restoring bodily health. Diet might not adequately nourish the body if the nervous system isn't working properly and getting the nutrients to the right places. Consequently, extra-dietary treatment is sometimes very helpful for enabling a wholesome diet to give its utmost benefit.

Good extra-dietary treatment is that which works *with* what God created into our bodies and into nature. Just as a natural diet will use little except plants and animals that grow on God's earth, chiropractic care uses little except a deep understanding of the interplay of the spinal cord, bones, muscles, and nerves of human beings. Many people have referred to allopathic treatment as sick-care rather than health-care, for the reason that it thrives on sickness rather than on health. Alternative treatment, however, thrives on wellness and prevention and on helping the body to function properly to prevent or slow disease. Additionally, alternative physicians, as they work with the body and with elements from God's creation, tend to use pure, natural methods of health promotion.

Natural healing in any of its numerous fields starts first with the fundamentals: working from the inside outward and addressing the root of the problem. Therefore, chiropractic work is a sensible field of natural healing. Chiropractic care lets the body function properly in order to heal itself properly. Natural and alternative health practitioners, by the way, have been subjected to the same bureaucratic and industry control that has hushed the health claims of natural foods and has squandered the freedoms of farmers and consumers. As a result, many people have never heard of these doctors or have only heard misinformation, which has given alternative doctors a bad reputation.

Like the quotation at the beginning of this chapter indicates, good doctors should be educating their patients on how the human body operates and how our bodies can be cared for in the best way possible. The word "doctor" originally comes from the Latin word meaning "to teach." The best doctors, then, will empower their patients with knowledge about the issues at hand. In my experience, naturopathic and chiropractic doctors have been more likely to expound on data for the benefit of the patient, though there are countless allopathic doctors and nurses with a deep understanding of the restoration of health. I believe that any doctors who understand preventative treatment for the human body have much wisdom and therefore much to teach.

Nutritional healing encompasses many different approaches. The nutritional method of healing ailments and diseases considers deficiencies and reactions that have arisen in the body. By testing blood, analyzing hair, or taking pH samples, natural practitioners will notice nutritional deficiencies, imbalanced hormones, or unnatural reactions and seek to remedy those rather than covering them up with drugs. Naturopathic doctors, for instance, might prescribe a certain supplement, a change in diet, or a kind of food, herbal extract, mineral compound, essential oil, or flower essence to apply to the body or take regularly. Natural foods can be applied medicinally in concentrated form as well as comprising a whole diet. Additionally, many institutes and programs exist to promote and facilitate the healing of degenerative diseases through natural methods.

Supplements are a highly promoted part of a healthy diet. From vitamins, herbs, root and leaf extracts, oils, and protein powders, there is a plethora of products on the market. Each family should study for themselves or consult a natural health practitioner concerning how much preventative medicine they want to use, taking into account their specific health and lifestyle needs. It is hard to receive adequate amounts of vitamins and minerals from our foods, however, so a basic whole-food vitamin and mineral supplement is a wise choice and will help prevent imbalances of single vitamins or minerals. Research where the nutrients are coming from to make sure they are from live and natural sources, not from synthetic sources as are some generic brands.

Nutritional supplements are for supplementing, or adding, to the diet and for building immunity. Numerous doctors in the books I have cited say that only minimal supplementation will be needed with a proper diet. Supplementing cannot make a bigger impact than the diet does. In other words, adding vitamins and supplements will not compensate for an improper diet. The majority of food intake needs to be healthy, with supplements taken primarily to augment certain areas that are already promoted to health by good foods.

To give an idea of the supplementing possibilities available, *The Maker's Diet* mentions a green super-food blend; a living, whole food supplement; cod liver oil; a fiber blend; coconut oil; protein powder; and aromatherapy.[3] *Nourishing Traditions* mentions, to name a few things, acerola berry (a super-fruit) powder, azomite mineral powder, bee pollen, blue-green algae, bitter herbs, high-vitamin butter, cod liver oil, colostrum, kelp, wheat germ oil, and probiotics.[4] Consult a naturopathic doctor, a chiropractor, or some of these books for specific recommendations.

Another element to health is *exercise*. Exercise is very important to get the body moving, improve circulation, and strengthen the heart, lungs, and other muscles. Walking is an excellent and relatively easy form of exercise. Doctors recommend walking for twenty minutes five days a week; thirty minutes three to four times a week; or an hour three times a week. Normal outdoor labor also accomplishes a similar benefit as walking does. Aerobic exercise is beneficial and cleansing for the body, especially when done for long enough to raise the heart rate and induce perspiration. Weight-lifting can also be quite beneficial both for muscle strengthening and weight loss, and there are many books that teach proper methods.

In *Living by Design*, Dr. Ray Strand shares some wisdom learned not in medical school but from experience and, it would seem, thoughtful observation in the school of God's creation. Most doctors are still doing what he did for twenty-three years: following the teachings from medical school and ignoring the place of nutrition, exercise, rest, and supplements.

> God has created the body with a tremendous ability to protect and heal itself, and the absolute best way to optimize the God-given natural defense systems is by eating a healthy diet, exercising consistently, resting in the Lord, and taking high-quality nutritional supplements. This is in stark contrast to what I learned in medical school and it is very different from what I told my patients for over 23 years.[5]

Yet another support to health is restful *sleep*—something that Americans get far too little of. The average adult sleeps for six or seven hours per night with many people getting only four or five hours of sleep. We should optimally have at least eight hours of sleep per night. Melatonin and prolactin are hormones that take eight or nine hours of sleep to produce, and they are necessary for a properly-functioning immune system.

When our ancestors, without electricity, went to bed with the sun and rose with the sun, they enjoyed the optimum amount of sleep. Today, however, with electric lights to provide perpetual daytime (and prevent melatonin production) and with carbohydrates that supply energy for people's midnight activities, we are totally out of tune with the biological rhythms that God created into nature and into our bodies. Researchers have found that if people eat carbohydrates—energy fuel—when they should normally be sleeping, the body stores them up in preparation for the expected "winter." Before the modern age, people would normally eat more carbohydrates in the summer and more protein in the winter due to seasonal availability. If we eat carbohydrates all year long and all night long, our bodies do not require such quantity so they store it up as extra fat. "The lower the number of hours you sleep, the higher the likelihood you will put on extra weight."[6]

In *The Maker's Diet,* Dr. Jordan Rubin refers to sleep as the "most important non-nutrient." He also believes that the body's natural rhythms are supported when people lay down and rise according to the daily cycles of the sun—as people did through history until the time of the Industrial Revolution.[7]

> Sleep may well be the single most important ingredient for digestive health. And it is important to get enough sleep at the right time. Some researchers believe that every minute you sleep before midnight is the equivalent of four minutes of sleep after midnight. Restful sleep will do wonders for your digestion and overall health.[8]

His note of *when* the most beneficial sleep occurs (before midnight) goes against the grain of our restless and overwhelmingly busy society, but it is worth heeding. With a little self-discipline, people can get several hours of deep sleep before midnight and wake early and refreshed for a productive morning. Certainly, social schedules occasionally demand late nights, but making a habit of getting "enough sleep at the right time" will make strides toward good health.

As Christians form an understanding of how God intended our bodies to operate, we should realize that food, exercise, sleep, and proper care can supply everything we need—as they have for millennia. For all of history, there have been doctors and other persons interested in studying health and in caring for sick and troubled persons, but multi-billion dollar hospital complexes are relatively recent innovations that came along directly with lifestyle changes in the habits of Western Civilization.

Healthful habits should always be our first choice—whether for living healthfully, or for healing an existing disease. Even if a drastic, conventional approach needs to be taken to counteract a health issue (surgery to remove a tumor, for instance), healthful habits and non-invasive techniques can only help in the healing process and in future prevention. Many people are able to manage chronic conditions and alleviate disease symptoms by following a wholesome diet and seeking natural care from health professionals. God's natural ways are always right and proper, whether they heal, or help to heal, a crisis in our bodies. Natural foods are our best medicine and our best prevention. God-given needs such as exercise and sleep are important in a healthful lifestyle, and alternative methods of disease prevention and healing are advantageous for whole-body health.

Chapter Twenty-four

Putting It into Practice

"She is like the merchants' ships; she bringeth her food from afar. She riseth also while it is yet night, and giveth meat to her household, and a portion to her maidens. She considereth a field, and buyeth it: with the fruit of her hands she planteth a vineyard."

—Psalm 31:14–16

IN THIS CHAPTER, I candidly share some actions my family has chosen to implement, not because I think these ideas are the right way for everyone, but to give encouragement and make the principles more personal.

Our own family's journey toward healthful, nutritious eating is one that started many years ago. Both of my parents grew up in California cities in families with mothers who cooked, but who generally cooked typical American foods: bacon and eggs for breakfast, sandwiches for lunch, meat and potatoes for dinner. Growing older, my parents were influenced by all that California had to offer—from the ocean, cropland, vineyards, and orchards. After they were married, they moved to Montana. Once here, they did more to supply their own food—hunting, fishing, gardening, and even beekeeping.

My mom has always loved to cook for our family—including making food from scratch and making a variety of ethnic foods. Our table was always spread with abundance, and guests acclaimed her tasty meals. She taught me to cook from the earliest age, and I have since enjoyed experimenting with natural ingredients and using her instruction as a foundation for exploring the culinary arts.

We have tried to "retake the control," or at least the knowledge, regarding our food. Knowledge, understanding, and wisdom are biblical virtues, and when we can exercise those virtues in the area of food, our families will be better off. Given that, the omniscience that Michael Pollan describes is a worthy goal:

> As cook in your kitchen, you enjoy an omniscience about your food that no amount of supermarket study or label reading could hope to match. Having retaken control of the meal from the food scientists and processors, you know exactly what is and is not in it...[1]

My mom's and my love of from-scratch cooking, as well as the acquisition of twenty acres which afforded the opportunity to be slightly more self-sustaining, was the beginning of our journey toward better nutrition. Until then (when my brother and I were eight and ten), we had eaten typical things: fast food, desserts, candy, etc. However, starting to tend our own property was a major step toward more understanding. We started to raise our own cattle to supply ourselves with beef. (This development took me a while to get used to; I had grown up eating venison and pronghorn antelope, and we still do.) Wanting the beef to be natural and grass-fed, got us thinking about chicken, too. While we never raised our own chickens, we started buying pasture-raised poultry. We would get organic turkeys for Thanksgiving, and those turkeys are so moist and flavorful that the tender slices hardly need to be topped with the usual assortment of jelly, gravy, and dressing used to make dry, conventional turkeys palatable.

My family grew a large garden which supplied us with vegetables, berries, and herbs until the next harvest. Our greenhouse boasted a jungle of tomato and cucumber vines and pepper and tomatillo plants. As we observed the growth of seeds, and tried saving seeds for planting the next year, we learned about genetically modified seeds (hybrids), which will not grow if replanted. Having our own produce helped us to incorporate it into more meals than was our normal habit. For a while, we had beehives that produced so much that we still have honey five years later. With our own pure, raw honey that we extracted and bottled ourselves, we started using it in baking and not just for tea and toast.

I enjoyed pondering biblical references to the cultivation of gardens and to the fruitfulness of the land. God, in His Word, uses botanical growth as an example of many things and even of extended judgment or increased blessing in the yield of crops.[2] In the time of the kings and prophets, there was apparently no such thing as highly-processed food and grocery corporations to serve as an alternative to private farms, yet God evidently looked with much favor upon the close involvement of raising the food we consume.

As we started to supply a large quantity of our food naturally (produce and meat), we reasonably began to think about the health of the rest of the things we ate. Similar to our family and other families learning about distinctively Christian education, we noticed one thing after another in our diet that was less-than-desirable. When we decide to pursue a healthier lifestyle, we will have to rid ourselves of all the baggage that we acquire while being influenced by the world.

We started grinding our own wheat from a local farm and canning our own applesauce with apples picked from a nearby homestead. While learning about all aspects of our diet was gradual, one new concept always led to another and our eyes were opened to yet another change we should make. We started reading the ingredients of everything we bought. If our home-grown food was so natural, it would be inconsistent to buy food full of artificial or impure ingredients. If white flour is unhealthy, white rice must be too, we thought. If we are cooking with better oils at home, we figured we needed to be careful about the oils in any store-bought baked goods. If we make whole-wheat pizza crust, we want the toppings to be natural and wholesome, lest it defeat the purpose of having a whole-wheat crust.

We stopped eating pork, corn syrup, canola oil, and white sugar. Beef, honey, olive oil, and evaporated cane crystals have replaced them. We stopped using aluminum cookware, conventional nonstick cookware, and microwaves, and learned to use stainless steel and toaster ovens or the stovetop. We learned to substitute the healthy version of ingredients into existing recipes, to cut back on sugar, and to add nutritious ingredients like wheat germ and herbs. I wish white flour was no longer in the house, but we hardly ever use it. I keep experimenting with baked goods using whole grain flours, and maybe my own home someday will be free of white ingredients—except coconut oil, of course.

Everyone else's journey will look different. Each family decides for themselves whether to garden and hunt, or whether to buy organic vegetables and meats at a store or from local merchants. We transitioned over many years and are still learning—and there are many more-knowledgeable people to learn from and more stellar practices we could follow. Starting to make small steps—and taking the next important action—is the largest decision of all.

I have tried to train my appetite by conjuring an image of what a food does to me: margarine sticking to me inside, inferior-quality chocolate making my face break out, and more. This way of thinking helps me to not even want to eat some foods. If you know and tell yourself that something is unhealthy, the food will not taste as good as it used to.

Through the years at our beloved Camp Hills Farm, we learned from several friends who were faithful to share their gardening and culinary discoveries. In more recent years, countless ladies have encouraged me with their health-conscious lifestyles and their wealth of health-oriented knowledge. The more I study, the more I am amazed at how intricately food nourishes us, and it is amazing that we don't have to make eating properly our life work. Certainly, many people do have the calling to study health in order to benefit mankind and better understand God's creation. More broadly speaking, however, God has already done all the work by creating good food and giving us directions on eating it. For instance, a knowledgeable nutritionist might study the copious health benefits of garlic and which ailments it can alleviate, but God has made garlic palatable to us and we can be assured that, since God made it, it is full of wonderful benefits whether we understand them or not.

Researching for this book has kept me learning more and more, and I just learned a lesson about applying my own principles better. While I know that organic meat is best, sometimes we buy non-organic fish. I know wild-caught fish is best, but the tilapia we have in our freezer was farm-raised. Well, I just read an article which said that farmed tilapia are given a hormone-altering drug that changes the sex of fish to male so that they are all the same size. This drug is toxic to the human liver, and the European Union has outlawed its use. If I had kept with the standard of either organically-grown or wild-caught fish, this mistake would have been avoided. This lesson demonstrates that applying principles can lead us wisely, even if we don't yet know all the facts. The fact that there exists the allowance and propensity for farmers to give drugs to farmed fish means that farmers likely will do so at some point, and we should avoid conventionally-farmed fish even if we do not know all the details.

With a little of my family's story shared, I will distill it here into principles to remember. Once you've understood the purpose of eating healthfully and have determined to do it, where should you start?

- First, try to streamline everything you cook with ingredients that are all-natural. Know exactly what you have in your pantry, refrigerator, and freezer. If a food or product is unhealthy, decide how bad it is and whether it is worth keeping. The health dangers of some things might not be worth the money spent on them. Or, use up the container and make an effort to buy a better brand or type on the next shopping trip. As you shop, read the ingredients on the labels of everything and resolve to buy clean and wholesome food—to let nothing unhealthy infiltrate your house. Eliminate all artificial and chemical additives and all pesticide-laden produce if possible.

At some point, people determine a standard for everything, regarding what will be allowed. Wise parents will guard the types of media that their children read and listen to; wise mothers will guard the types of food that enter the cabinet—and then the children's mouths.

- As you get better at reading labels and guarding ingredients, the next concept to consider is whether the processing is wholesome. The process involved could apply to meat, milk, and eggs, as has been discussed previously, but what is really meant here is packaged food. Sure, you can get an "organic" granola bar that is still loaded with organic white sugar, organic white flour, and organic soybean oil, all diminishing the benefits from the rolled oats, or you could get a heartier bar made with organic oats and dried fruit and sweetened with applesauce or brown rice syrup. The foods with the simplest ingredients and simplest preparations will usually be the most wholesome. Be warned: all-natural foods can still have bad kinds of fats, sugars, or other ingredients (canola, soy, etc.). Be discriminating in your selection. Eat the right—the good—kinds of each and every type of food. Making your own foods from scratch with the proper ingredients is the best way to ensure the food's healthfulness.

- At this point, you may also start thinking about where you buy your food. Local food will be the freshest and purchasing it will support the local economy rather than a far-away city. Farmers' markets and roadside stands are good places to get fresh produce and homemade food products. There are grains and meats raised naturally in almost every region or at least distributed by small regional companies. If you are in need of some prepared foods, buy organic versions at the local grocery store and this will encourage stores to carry more organic food.

- Once you have honed down the kinds of foods that you will be cooking with, match them together in the right proportions for nutritious meals. Generally, we need fewer carbohydrates than Americans typically eat, and instead, a variety of more clean proteins and fibrous fruits and vegetables both raw and cooked. You might have all the right alternative ingredients for making less-refined and low-sugar desserts, but wholesome desserts should still be an occasional treat, not a twice-daily occurrence.

To boil down this list:

1. Use pure, natural ingredients.
2. Employ wholesome processes.
3. Balance nutrient proportions.

Know the origin of every box, bag, bottle, carton, and can that goes from the field to the factory to your feast-table. Know, and be satisfied with, how food was grown, how it was made ready for consumption and packaging, and how it should be incorporated into your meals. The more you study health, the more the principles will become ingrained, and terms such as "natural," "pure," "super-food," "vitamin-rich," and "wholesome" will be on your mind as you shop for and prepare meals for your family. The more progress you make toward healthy choices, the more exciting, and hopefully less-overwhelming, meal preparation will become.

It seems to me that looking for wholesome food is something of a treasure hunt; it has to be carefully sought, and it's a prize once you find it. The fact that pure food is uncommon but valuable makes looking for it an adventure—and finding it, a delight. Searching for good food is satisfying and rewarding, and making a few discoveries spurs the seeker on toward more discoveries. Won't you try it? I think you'll be pleasantly surprised at how exciting it is to find restaurants, magazines, friends, and especially food that promotes natural health!

Author Jonny Bowden states the following lesson in his book *The 150 Healthiest Foods on Earth*, a volume where he reveals exactly what kind of "quality" and "real" foods we should be eating.

> Despite the best efforts of the food industry to make us think our food just magically somehow appears in the supermarket aisle, our food actually comes from somewhere. And where it comes from— where and how it grows in the case of plants and what it eats and how it was raised in the case of animals—has a lot to do with its quality. So let's start with a basic premise: *The quality of the food we eat comes from the quality of the food our food eats...*
>
> What you eat probably doesn't ultimately matter as much as how much processing it's undergone. Real food—whole food with minimal processing—contains a virtual pharmacy of nutrients, phytochemicals, enzymes, vitamins, minerals, antioxidants, anti-inflammatories, and healthful fats, and can keep you alive and thriving into your tenth decade.[3]

Our food has eaten food, so if we want to know what we are eating, we will need to know what our food has eaten. That, my friends, is the stuff of life and health.

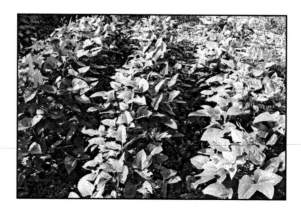

Chapter Twenty-five

Questions to Ponder

"If by gaining knowledge we destroy our health, we labour
for a thing that is useless in our hands."[1]

—John Locke

AS I COME toward the close of this book, I want to submit several questions to help
you gauge what you have hopefully gleaned. Below is a list in which I sought to
address many of the themes discussed so far.

- Have I renewed my interest in God's creation and my interest in causing my use
  of creation to reflect His goodness and provision?
- Have I come to view my food purchasing and preparation as an avenue of furthering
  godly culture in my home and glorifying Him thereby?

And he said unto them, "When ye pray, say, Our Father which art in heaven, Hallowed
be thy name. Thy kingdom come. Thy will be done, as in heaven, so in earth. Give us
day by day our daily bread..."

—Luke 11:2–3

- Have I understood that diet is the number one factor that contributes to our
  health, whether for the better or for the worse?
- Have I understood that the general health of Americans has terribly deteriorated
  in the last several generations as God's ways have been neglected, but that health

can be regained for ours and future generations by returning to His ways, which are also the ways of our ancestors?

- Have I asked God to give our family wisdom in selecting our course, to give us mercy as we fail, to give us health as we obey His principles, and to give us humility as we continue learning?
- Have I, as a woman, sought and taken responsibility to nourish my family with healthful foods and sought to maintain my own health for the nurturing of children?
- Alternately, have I, as a man, sought and taken responsibility to direct my family, including children, to a wholesome lifestyle and sought to provide the resources to do so?
- Have I formed convictions about our family's diet, after thoughtful research, and determined to deferentially follow these standards whenever possible?
- Have we, as parents, taught our children what we believe about God's creation, earthly stewardship, individual responsibility, and principles of nutrition so that they will pursue healthful choices with their own families in the future?
- Have I come to view conventional food and medicine with reservation and to accept organic foods and preventative care as my best source of sustenance and healing?
- Have I purged our cupboards to remove undesirable items and replaced them with the culinary treasures of historical renown and vibrant nutrition?
- Have I considered my grocery budget with regard to convenience foods, conventional foods, natural foods, homemade foods, and local foods in relation to how they will nourish and whom they will subsidize?
- Have I determined to make immediate changes to my meals rather than putting this and other health-related books back on the shelf and giving no lasting heed to their message?
- "Today, which food system advanced because of me—farm friendly food or industrial food?" asks Mr. Salatin.[2] Or, as corollaries to that question: Today, was disease invited or prevented by my eating habits? Was health promoted or inhibited by my lifestyle habits?

I would like to summarize two contrasting ideas. Everything formed at the time of creation by our sovereign God has the history of the world behind it and is perpetually reliable for the increase of wise and godly culture by mankind. Everything formulated by finite human beings in the last couple of centuries has little history behind it and has the precarious potential to decrease the strength of mankind's culture if used unwisely.

If my readers have understood the contrast between the design, record, and usage of natural versus unnatural foods and products, *Health for Godly Generations* will not have been written in vain. You have not read this book in vain if you generate changes in your lifestyle and reform the way you think about our Western Civilization. I hope that the care and concern with which you start to approach your health will eventually lead to delight as you take dominion *coram deo*—under God— over this area of your life.

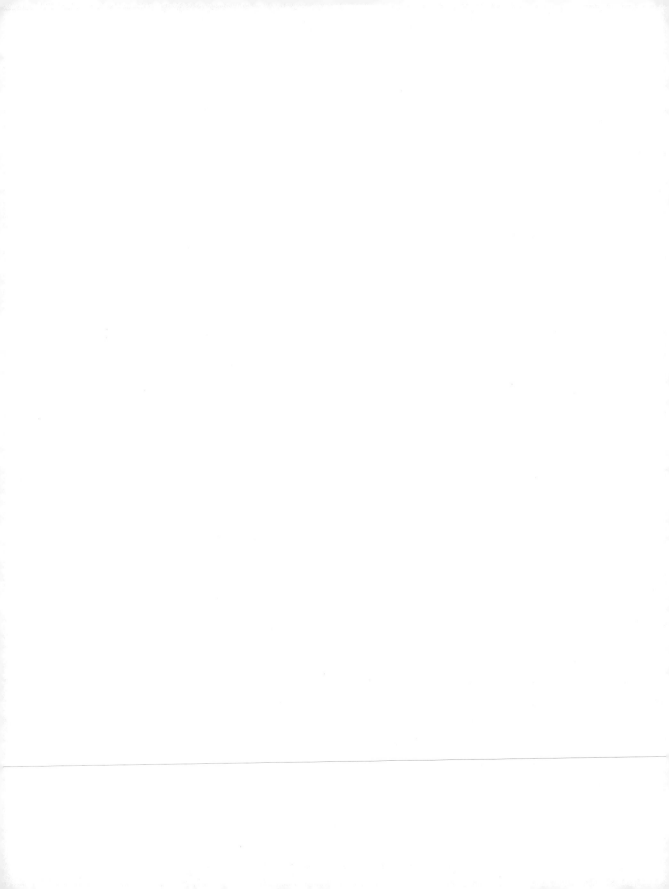

Chapter Twenty-six

Resources for Further Study

"...Of making many books there is no end; and much study is a weariness of the
flesh. Let us hear the conclusion of the whole matter: Fear God, and keep his
commandments: for this is the whole duty of man."

—Ecclesiastes 12:12–13

DURING THE TIME I have been writing this book, I continually came across more
and more books that appear to be excellent reading material. I could have kept
studying and adding to this book, but then it would never have been published. Eventually
I had to stop and think, "Here—this is the material I want to share with my friends and
other Christians." The books that I keep finding only confirm the principles that I have
addressed here, and I trust that your further study will do the same if you approach it
wisely. Multitudes of books are on the market for further research, and I look forward to
reading more. I always like to find more tidbits of data that demonstrate God's wonderful
works in creation and history. I know I am going to continue my own research in order
to invest in my life and the lives of my future family, if God so ordains, and I hope you
will, too.

When researching, consider the source that the information is coming from. You
can find an article on just about anything from any number of perspectives—in books,
industry publications, or on the internet. However, you should take everything with a
grain of salt, as the saying goes. For example, while Polynesian peoples have thrived on
coconut oil for centuries, the soy industry has, in the last fifty years, started saying that
coconut oil is bad and that people should eat soybean oil instead. Ask yourself, is the

record of history supporting a specific nutrition claim, or is a company with little history making the supposed claim? Consider who is telling you something, how long they have been saying it, and what their agenda is.

In your research, you might notice a seeming discrepancy. Seeing problems with conventionally-grown meat, various trustworthy sources of health information recommend a more grain-based diet. Other trustworthy sources, noticing problems with refined flour products, recommend a more meat-based diet. Both respected schools of thought make good observations and claim great results. However, *whole* grains are very nutritious and *organic* meat and dairy products have historically been consumed in great quantity. The key is keeping meats and grains in their wholesome forms and combining them with vegetable-based proteins and carbohydrates, while understanding that certain body types may require greater or smaller proportions of protein and carbohydrates. People also have varying nutritional needs based on past or present health conditions.

Many books appear to give similar ideas as each other. After all, wisdom is wisdom, and believing the right principles will lead to similar conclusions. Scientific research with a bent toward acknowledging health, history, and longevity consistently points to the wisdom of God's design and His ways. My purpose in the last few chapters has been to synthesize many of the themes found in my research and to give, I hope, specific dietary suggestions adequate for fleshing out the principles in the first few chapters. Many of the books and websites I used in recent research are listed in the following bibliography. I have quoted from some well-respected sources, but there are many, many other doctors teaching the same truths about real food and healing medicine. To delve into more research, find a few of the books listed, find other books by the same authors, read the books recommended in these books, or read material by the people who endorse these books.

If you are skeptical about the research for, as an example, cell phones, chemicals, caffeine, alcohol, or anything else I gave cautions about, read the work of health-minded medical doctors either in their books or on their websites. This is highly recommended; there was no way I could document or wanted to document thorough evidence for these issues. If you want to know interesting facts such as why inflammation causes disease, what causes oxidative stress, how much more calcium is in watercress than in milk, what properties in oranges fight infection, or which properties of oranges strengthen the capillaries, read some of the following books!

Start, or continue, your healthful lifestyle by eating and using good and natural foods and other household products. Find material that speaks to your personal needs or interests. If you want to know more, for instance, about gluten-free diets, low-glycemic diets, Mediterranean-type diets, or about apple cider vinegar, raw milk, or coconut oil, find a book on it. Knowledge will encourage and inspire.

Listed below are some of my favorite resources, so far—and the most inspiring, though I do not agree with everything they say (and they might not agree with everything I say). The subject which my book has merely been able to introduce is ably expanded by these selected books as well as others in the bibliography.

- *Nourishing Traditions* by Sally Fallon
- *Living By Design* by Dr. Ray Strand and Bill Ewing
- *Body By God* by Dr. Ben Lerner
- *What the Bible Says about Healthy Living* by Dr. Rex Russell
- *Patient, Heal Thyself* by Dr. Jordan Rubin
- *The Maker's Diet* by Dr. Jordan Rubin
- *The French Diet* by Michel Montignac
- *The Coconut Oil Miracle* by Bruce Fife
- *In Defense of Food* by Michael Pollan
- *The 150 Healthiest Foods on Earth* by Jonny Bowden
- *What You Don't Know May Be Killing You* by Dr. Don Colbert
- *Holy Cows and Hog Heaven* by Joel Salatin
- *Food, Inc.* (film) by Robert Kenner and Eric Schlosser
- *Home Safe Home* by Debra Lynn Dadd
- *The Organic Food Guide* by Steve Meyerowitz
- *Total Health Program* by Dr. Joseph Mercola
- *Creation Regained* by Albert Wolters

Whole-food cookbooks abound, but I only have a handful. One good thing about whole-food cookbooks and vegetarian cookbooks is that they tend to showcase vegetables and fruit and use them more creatively, and more substantively, than most cookbooks. In the past, my mother and I have adapted good quality gourmet recipes (such as Williams-Sonoma®, America's Test Kitchen™, or Barefoot Contessa™) by substituting alternate ingredients where present, such as using cane juice crystals in place of white sugar, whole wheat pastry flour instead of white flour, or olive oil instead of vegetable oil. I mention this so that cooking with healthy foods does not sound too intimidating. It can be rather simple if you have the right ingredients and right motives.

On the other hand, cooking is an art that is almost limitless in its possibilities of precision and imagination. One of my personal aspirations is to become more proficient in baking with soaked whole grains and in cooking with seasonal foods, local foods, super-foods, and fermented foods. The meals that currently grace our table—in case you happen to see—often look like normal homemade meals, but you can be assured that the ingredients are of a fine and natural quality. It is my mission, though, to make more whole-food style meals that look atypical but taste delicious. I want to encourage people that eating for nutrition is invigorating both to the mind and the body.

Whether from reading, cooking, hiking, or gardening, becoming more aware of the wonders of God's world is very enlightening. It is the privilege of "all people that on earth do dwell"[1] to discover how perfectly God created the natural environment to sustain abundant life.

Abundant life: this is what Christians have been given spiritually and eternally by virtue of the saving mercy of the Lord Jesus Christ. Our physical lives as stewards over God's earth will be, likewise, more abundant if they are lived through the lens of our redeemed standing in Christ. Man's ways are pitiful and fleeting, but God's ways are abundant and everlasting.

May all of our research cause us to fall more in love with our Savior who transforms hearts and minds and reforms lives and cultures. May our distinct and purposeful lifestyles be a display of heart and health reformation. May the Church's journey on this earth give Him all the glory and all the praise; He hath done wondrous things! Our Lord said, "I am come that they might have life, and that they might have it more abundantly" (John 10:10).

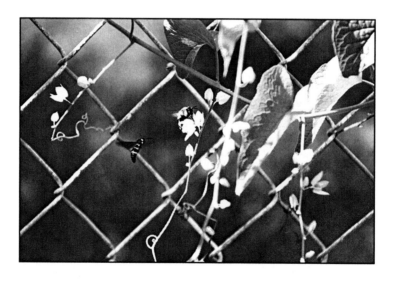

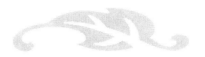

Appendix A:
Creation versus Evolution

EVERY CHAPTER IN this book is built on the presupposition that the Lord Jesus Christ created all things in heaven and on earth. In six twenty-four hour days, He made light and darkness, land and water, stars and planets, plants and creatures, man and woman—out of nothing. It was all very good.

> He hath made the earth by his power, he hath established the world by his wisdom, and hath stretched out the heaven by his understanding.
>
> —Jeremiah 51:15

> In the beginning was the Word, and the Word was with God, and the Word was God. The same was in the beginning with God. All things were made by him; and without him was not any thing made that was made.
>
> —John 1:1–3

It is not my purpose here to give evidence for a defense of biblical creation against the theory of evolution, but I want to affirm the doctrine of creation as the basis for everything I wrote in this book. If Christians seek to believe the Bible as God's inerrant truth, and if Christians seek to obey God's will for their lives, then the Genesis account of creation must be the requisite starting point. Neither Darwinian evolution nor theistic evolution is compatible with the Genesis account. Scientific evidence, properly and logically explained, confirms the claim of the Lord Jesus Christ as Creator of the world.

If the earth and mankind slowly evolved from a primordial pond via "intermediate forms," then death is to be hoped for because it brings progress. If plants and animals—our food sources—slowly evolved, then people have no basis for determining whether natural foods are any better than the manufactured foods of man's recent technological "progress."

However, if the earth and mankind were divinely created out of nothing in six days, then death brings sorrow because sin was the first thing to bring ruin to God's world. If plants and animals were created to further the life and work of mankind, then people do have a basis for studying the healthiest, most natural foods for the benefit of society.

Believing in the creation account in Genesis is foundational and essential for everything else that Christians believe. *The Lie: Evolution* by Ken Ham is a very powerful text for explaining that creation is fundamental to the Gospel of Jesus Christ and other Christian beliefs. I also encourage my readers to study resources from Answers in Genesis and the Institute for Creation Research or other creation organizations if you question creation's validity or sensibility for either science or the Christian faith.

Knowing God's work of creation must come before any study of man's purpose on earth, lest the latter be futile. We must know where life, mankind, food, and death came from before we can understand the food that best protects and promotes man's life. I hope that you will have faith in the inspired Word of God from Genesis to Revelation, for it is only then that Christians can approach and apply principles for wholesome health.

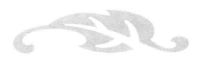

Appendix B:
From My Journal

EVIDENTLY FALTERING BUT searching for clarity, the following journal entries about nutrition were penned in the volume I filled during my father's sickness, five winters before the publication of this book. Weak despair of where to find good advice conflicted with a strong desire to change our eating habits. At the time of these journal entries, my family and I were introduced to the idea of eating all raw, vegetarian foods, yet I was fearful of how unconventional this would be. There are many truths in the following paragraphs as well as many things I still needed to learn. That season of life—and death—got my attention, never to be released.

I learned that nutrition is not something that can be sprinkled on your food, but must constitute a whole lifestyle. I learned that we should not presume upon health. I learned to respect the world's cuisines in their pure, traditional, and wholesome forms. I learned that one can still enjoy cooking, eating, and serving natural foods. I have come to a more balanced perspective on diet, I trust, and now have a better message to share with other Christians—the message contained in this book. However, I share the following thoughts to show what it was like to be confronted with the issue of health, and to be thrust toward wanting answers.

Many people we know are doing fine on normal cuisine, but so were we until this happened with Dad. We have long known that nutrition is inextricably linked to physical function, but how much attention should we give to it? If we ate only fresh fruit and vegetables, maybe we would have added energy and perfect digestion. I think there is a point where preserving one's health overwhelms the benefits gained from it. I do not think we are nearly to that point yet, so we'll have to change some things.

Oh, I pray for wisdom. How much do we use the knowledge God has given us without being paranoid or legalistic? I pray for answers. I pray that my family now, and my future family someday, can be sensitive to diet and nutrition—not so ignorant as to eat unhealthfully, but not so strict that we can't enjoy the products of a land that "flows with milk and honey," as was the land God gave to the Israelites.

Of course, what is 'healthful' is very subjective. To some it means occasionally including an apple along with whatever junk food you eat; to some it means having a token serving of overcooked vegetables at every dinner; to others it means only vegan foods; to others it means making raw juice five times a day. What seems healthful to one person is forbidden by another. I pray that we can use our education and resources to prepare nourishing food while not inhibiting our giving and partaking of hospitality and of the other tasks God has given us.

I was thinking about nutrition again and I don't know what to do. I don't want to feel guilty about eating certain things, like at our friends' house last night. Yet, I want to make use of the knowledge God gives us. If God really intended for the food-combining diet to be followed [such as not eating protein and starches together], why don't any world cuisines follow these principles? I'm sure our family is far from the maximum possible health, but the rest of us, other than Dad, are strong. How involved should we get in pursuing healthful foods?

I guess my fear is the demise of my love of cooking. I like combining as many different things as possible, to add flavor, texture, color, and variety. I like presenting a display of choices at special occasions. And now we hear that a person should eat only a handful of carefully matched ingredients at a time. [Simple foods, and the avoidance of heavy protein and starch in equal proportion, are still a good idea for aiding digestion, however.] I want to do right and not ignore something that has merit. I think of how my friends and future family will like to eat, and I want food to be appealing to them.

I don't want cooking to be a source of worry. I used to think that I loved cooking to feed my family and friends and that I loved to cook with healthful ingredients and be creative in the kitchen. But now that is all challenged. Now almost every day we are bombarded with information: "Eat this to prevent cancer;" "To aid digestion, omit this food;" "For healthy skin, you need this;" "Take this to fix this;" "Exercise now to prevent disease later;" "Bodies deteriorate with this kind of food." Everyone wants to scare you into something and make you spend money, but nobody has all the answers or the perfect diet. There is a fine line between eating to be full, enjoying the art of eating good food, and really watching what one consumes and taking time to improve health. It is almost despairing trying to figure it out.

I had wanted, once, to write a book about nutrition, but now I have hardly any answers myself. Is it healthier to dwell so much on what food we take in, or spend that time working? We could spend all day eating in separate courses for improved digestion and making juice several times a day—but I don't know if it is worth it. But then I look at my Dad rapidly declining unless the Lord intervenes, and it makes me believe that improving health is worthwhile. I will someday be responsible, other than a husband's direction, for my future family's nutrition and well-being, and I need to know how to approach that responsibility. I think we can prevent chronic disease by what we eat. I see so many people struggling with their health and living with complications, and I don't want anyone I know to turn out that way again if I can help it.

So, thankful for my own health, prompted to find answers, and desirous to prevent illness, I set out to study, and have been studying ever since. At one point, I became so concerned with the physical state of people around us, and their lack of awareness about food, that I knew I had to write this book—and the Lord gave more wisdom than I clearly had as I wrote in my journal five years ago.

It was challenging to write this book, because I think some might feel that it suppresses the lifestyle of relatively healthy people. However, the minute I hear of yet another person struggling with their health, I am again convinced that the message needed to be written. By His grace, the information in this book will help someone. By His grace, I will seek to follow principles of health to the best of my ability, yet remain humble and rely on His strength alone for His glory alone.

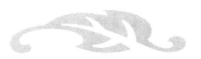

Bibliography

Bauman, Edward. *Eating for Health*. Penngrove, Calif.: Bauman College, 2008.

Bauman, Edward. *Recipes and Remedies for Rejuvenation*. Penngrove, Calif.: Bauman College, 2005.

Balch, James F. and Phyllis A. *Prescription for Nutritional Healing*. Second Edition. New York: Avery Publishing, 1997.

Balch, Phyllis A. *Prescription for Dietary Wellness*. Second Edition. New York: Avery Publishing, 2003.

Baxter, Richard. *A Christian Directory*. Volume I. Second Printing. Morgan, Penn.: Soli Deo Gloria, 2000.

Berthold-Bond, Annie. *Clean and Green*. Woodstock, New York: Ceres Press, 1994.

Bollinger, Ty. "A Cancer Epidemic." Home School Digest, Volume 17 Number 4. Covert, Mich.: 2007.

Bowden, Jonny, Ph.D, CNS. *The 150 Healthiest Foods on Earth*. Beverly, Mass.: Fair Winds Press, 2007.

Campbell, Diane. *Step-by-Step to Natural Food*. Clearwater, Flor.: CC Publishers, 1979.

Colbert, Don M.D. *What Would Jesus Eat?* Nashville: Nelson Books, 2002.

Colbert. Don M.D. *What You Don't Know May Be Killing You!* Lake Mary, Flor.: Siloam Press, 2000.

Cox, Janice. *Natural Beauty at Home*. New York: Henry Holt, 1995.

Cummins, Ronnie and Ben Lilliston. *Genetically Engineered Food*. New York: Marlowe and Company, 2000.

Dadd, Debra Lynn. *Home Safe Home*. New York: Tarcher/Putnam, 1997.

Dufty, William. *Sugar Blues*. Reissue. New York: Grand Central Publishing, 1993.

Dye, Michael. *Vaccinations: Deception and Tragedy*. Shelby, North Carolina: Hallelujah Acres, 1999.

Fallon, Sally with Mary Enig. *Nourishing Traditions*. Revised Second Edition. Washington, D.C.: NewTrends Publishing, 2001.

Fife, Bruce. *The Coconut Oil Miracle*. New York: Avery, 2001.

Goldbeck, Nikki and David Goldbeck. *American Whole Foods Cuisine*. New York: Plume, 1983.

Graimes, Nicola. *Whole Foods Kitchen*. East Bridgewater, Mass.: World Publishing Group, 2008.

Griffin, G. Edward. *World Without Cancer*. Revised and updated edition. Westlake Village, Calif.: American Media, 1999.

Guttersen, Dr. Connie, R.D. PhD. *The Sonoma Diet*. Des Moines: Meredith Books, 2005.

Hellmiss, Margot. *Natural Healing with Apple Cider Vinegar*. New York: Sterling Publishing, 1998.

Henry, Matthew. *Matthew Henry's Commentary in One Volume*. Zondervan Classics Reference Series. Edited by Rev. Leslie Church. Grand Rapids: Zondervan, 1999.

Holy Bible, The. King James Version.

James, John Angell. *A Help to Domestic Happiness*. Reprinted. Morgan, Penn.: Soli Deo Gloria Publications, 1995.

Jehle, Dr. Paul. *Go Ye Therefore...And Teach All Nations*. Volume II. Columbus, Geor.: Brentwood Christian Press, 2007.

Kaufman, Donald G., and Cecilia M. Franz. *Biosphere 2000: Protecting our Global Environment*. Second Edition. Dubuque, Iowa: Kendall Hunt Publishing, 1996.

Kenner, Robert, producer. *Food, Inc*. DVD. Eric Schlosser, narrator. Magnolia Home Entertainment, 2008.

Kinderlehrer, Jane. *Confessions of a Sneaky Organic Cook*. Emmaus, Penn.: Rodale Press, 1971.

Kloss, Jethro. *Back to Eden*. Revised and Expanded Second Edition. Loma Linda, Calif.: Back to Eden Publishing, 1997.

Lerner, Dr. Ben. *Body By God*. Nashville: Thomas Nelson, 2003.

McDowell, Stephen, and Mark Beliles. *The American Dream: Jamestown and the Planting of the American Christian Republic*. Charlottesville, Virg.: Providence Foundation, 2007.

Meyerowitz, Steve. *Food Combining and Digestion*. Great Barrington, Mass.: Sproutman Publications, 2002.

Meyerowitz, Steve. *The Organic Food Guide.* Guilford, Conn.: Morris Book Publishing, 2004.

Mercola, Dr. Joseph with Bryan Vaszily, Dr. Kendra Pearsall, and Nancy Lee Bentley. *Dr. Mercola's Total Health Program.* Shaumberg, Ill.: Mercola.com, 2004.

Montignac, Michel. *The French Diet.* New York: DK Publishing, 2005.

Perry, Luddene with Dan Schultz. *A Field Guide to Buying Organic.* New York: Bantam Books, 2005.

Phillips, Douglas. *"How the Scots Saved Christendom."* Disk One. Audio CD series. San Antonio: Vision Forum Ministries, 2008.

Phillips, Douglas. *"The Family Table."* Audio CD series. San Antonio: Vision Forum Ministries, 2009.

Pollan, Michael. *In Defense of Food: An Eater's Manifesto.* New York: The Penguin Press, 2008.

Price, Weston A., DDS. *Nutrition and Physical Degeneration.* Eighth Edition. La Mesa, Calif.: The Price-Pottenger Nutrition Foundation, 2008.

Rondberg, Terry A., D.C. *Chiropractic First.* Chandler, Ariz.: The Chiropractic Journal, 1998.

Rubin, Dr. Jordan S. *Patient, Heal Thyself.* Eleventh Printing. Topanga, Calif.: Freedom Press, 2003.

Rubin, Dr. Jordan S. *The Maker's Diet.* New York: The Berkley Publishing Group, 2004.

Russell, Rex, M.D. *What the Bible Says About Healthy Living.* Ventura, Calif.: Regal Publishing, 1996.

Salatin, Joel. *Pastured Poultry Profits.* Swoope, Virg.: Polyface, Inc., 1999.

Salatin, Joel. *Salad Bar Beef.* Swoope, Virg.: Polyface, Inc., 1995.

Salatin, Joel. *Holy Cows and Hog Heaven.* Swoope, Virg.: Polyface, Inc., 2004.

Shahani, Khem, Ph.D. *Cultivate Health From Within.* Danbury, Connec.: Vital Health Publishing, 2005.

Strand, Dr. Ray and Bill Ewing with Todd Hillard *Living By Design.* Rapid City, S. Dak.: Real Life Press, 2006.

Strand, Ray D., M.D. *What Your Doctor Doesn't Know About Nutritional Medicine.* Nashville: Thomas Nelson, 2002.

Swan, Karey. *Hearth and Home.* Fourth Edition. Sisters, Ore.: Loyal Publishing, 1999.

Swanson, Kevin. *The Book of Psalms: The Heart of the Word.* Book I: Psalms 1–41. Parker, Colo.: Generations with Vision, 2008.

Swanson, Kevin. *Upgrade.* Nashville: Broadman & Holman, 2006.

Tannahill, Reay. *Food in History.* New and Revised Edition. New York: Crown Publishers, 1989.

Thrash, Agatha M.D. and Calvin Thrash, M.D. *Poison with a Capital C.* Seale, Alabama: NewLifestyle Books, 2000.

Tourles, Stephanie. *Organic Body Care Recipes*. North Adams, Mass.: Storey Publishing, 2007.

Trager, James. *The Food Chronology*. New York: Henry Holt, 1995.

Trudeau, Kevin. *Natural Cures "They" Don't Want You to Know About*. Updated Edition. Elk Grove Village, Ill.: Alliance Publishing Group, 2004.

Van Til, Henry R. *The Calvinistic Concept of Culture*. Grand Rapids: Baker Book House, 1959.

Wentz, Dr. Myron. *Invisible Miracles*. Rosarito Beach, Baja California: Medicis, S.C., 2002.

Westminster Confession of Faith. Reprinted. Glasgow, Scotland: Free Presbyterian Publications, 2003.

Wolcott, William and Trish Fahey. *The Metabolic Typing Diet*. New York: Broadway Books, 2002.

Wolters, Albert M. *Creation Regained*. Second Edition. Grand Rapids: Wm. B. Eerdmanns Publishing, 2005.

Woolley, Benjamin. *Heal Thyself*. New York: Harper Collins, 2004.

Suggested websites:

News and research:

Price-Pottenger Foundation	www.westonaprice.org
Dr. Mercola	www.drmercola.com
Natural News	www.naturalnews.com
Dr. Jordan Rubin	www.gardenoflife.com
World's Healthiest Foods	www.whfoods.org

Selected author websites:

Plymouth Rock Foundation	www.plymrock.org
Bruce Fife	www.coconutresearchcenter.org
Michel Montignac	www.montignac.com

Natural living and homemaking helps:

The Nourishing Gourmet	www.thenourishinggourmet.com
Passionate Homemaking	www.passionatehomemaking.com
Kitchen Stewardship	www.kitchenstewardship.com
Keeper of the Home	www.keeperofthehome.org

Please visit **www.healthforgenerations.com** for ordering and contact information for this book.

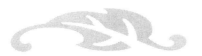

Endnotes

Introduction

1. William Dufty, *Sugar Blues*, pg. 49

Chapter One

1. Jakob Bernoulli, 17th century Swiss Mathematician
2. Westminster Confession of Faith, Of Providence, Chapter 5.2
3. Isaac Watts, "I Sing the Mighty Power of God"
4. Ray Strand and Bill Ewing, *Living By Design*, pg. 4
5. Eric Schlosser, Food Inc. film, interview of Joel Salatin

Chapter Two

1. John Calvin, Protestant theologian and reformer
2. Albert Wolters, *Creation Regained*, pg. 57
3. Ibid. pg. 49
4. Ibid. pg. 72
5. Maltbie D. Babcock, "This Is My Father's World"
6. Paul Jehle, *Go Ye Therefore…and Teach all Nations*, Volume Two, pp. 410–413
7. Kevin Swanson, *The Book of Psalms: The Heart of the Word*, Book I, pg. 18

Chapter Three

1. Joseph Wood Krutch, naturalist
2. Ray Strand and Bill Ewing, *Living By Design*, pg. 109
3. Ibid. pg. 122
4. Joseph Mercola, *Dr. Mercola's Total Health Program*, pg. 1
5. Ray Strand and Bill Ewing, *Living By Design*, pg. 140

Chapter Four

1. Jordan Rubin, *Patient, Heal Thyself*, pg. 113
2. Ibid. pg. 126
3. Ray Strand and Bill Ewing, *Living By Design*, pg. 131
4. Stephen McDowell and Mark Beliles, *The American Dream*, pg. 103
5. Ben Lerner, *Body By God*, pg. 13

Chapter Five

1. Mark Kurlansky, journalist
2. Michel Montignac, *The French Diet*, pg. 91
3. Don Colbert, *What You Don't Know May Be Killing You*, pg. 4
4. Ben Lerner, *Body By God*, pp. 26–27
5. Ray Strand and Bill Ewing, *Living By Design*, pg. xi
6. Sally Fallon, *Nourishing Traditions*, pg. 1
7. Herbert M. Shelton
8. Debra Lynn Dadd, *Home Safe Home*, pg. 214
9. Richard Baxter, *A Christian Dictionary*, Volume I, "Directions for governing taste and appetite," pg. 315

Chapter Six

1. Paul Jehle, *Go Ye Therefore...and Teach all Nations*, Volume Two, pg. 415
2. Westminster Confession of Faith, Chapter 3.1
3. Ibid. Chapter 5.2
4. Ray Strand and Bill Ewing, *Living by Design*, pg. 15
5. Ibid, pg. 125

Chapter Seven

1. Rudyard Kipling, English poet, "The Glory of the Garden"
2. from the Great Law of the Iroquois State
3. Paul Jehle, *Go Ye Therefore…and Teach All Nations*, Volume Two, pg. 413
4. Donald Kaufman and Cecilia Franz, *Biosphere 2000*, pp. 18–19
5. see *The American Dream*, Stephen McDowell and Mark Beliles, and *Of Plymouth Plantation* by William Bradford

Chapter Eight

1. Samuel Johnson, English essayist
2. Bruce Fife, *The Coconut Oil Miracle*, pg. 27
3. Joel Salatin, *Holy Cows and Hog Heaven*, pg. 84
4. Paul Jehle, *Go Ye Therefore…and Teach All Nations*, Volume Two, pg. 417
5. Ibid, pg. 419
6. Sally Fallon, *Nourishing Traditions*, pg. 22
7. Ray Strand and Bill Ewing, *Living By Design*, pg. 145

Chapter Nine

1. James Trager, *The Food Chronology*, year 1952
2. Eric Schlosser, Food Inc. film
3. Ibid.
4. Ty Bollinger, "A Cancer Epidemic," Home School Digest Volume 17 Number 4, pp. 45–46
5. Jordan Rubin, *Patient, Heal Thyself*, pg. 41
6. Paul Jehle, *Go Ye Therefore…and Teach All Nations*, Volume Two, pp. 423–424
7. Nicola Graimes, *Whole Foods Kitchen*, pg. 6
8. James Trager, *The Food Chronology*, years 1890–1895
9. Ibid, years 1940–1960
10. Matthew Henry, *Commentary in One Volume*, Ecclesiastes 7:10
11. Kevin Swanson, *Upgrade*, pg. 109
12. Doug Phillips, "How the Scots Saved Christendom," Disk One
13. Bruce Fife, *The Coconut Oil Miracle*, pg. 38
14. Ibid, pg. 8

Chapter Ten

1. Thomas Jefferson, U.S. President
2. Paul Jehle, *Go Ye Therefore...and Teach All Nations*, Volume Two, pg.425
3. Steve Meyerowitz, *The Organic Food Guide*, pg. 38
4. Ben Lerner, *Body by God*, pg. 41
5. Weston Price, *Nutrition and Physical Degeneration*, pg. 15
6. Ibid, pg. 3

Chapter Eleven

1. Jacques DeLangre, biochemist
2. Diane Campbell, *Step-by-Step to Natural Food*, pg. 4
3. Albert Wolters, *Creation Regained*, pg. 131
4. John Angell James, *Help for Domestic Happiness*, pp. 118–119
5. Michael Pollan, *In Defense of Food*, pg. 189
6. William Dufty, *Sugar Blues*, pg. 211
7. Joseph D. Beasley and Jerry J. Swift, quoted in *Nourishing Traditions*, pg. 370
8. Sally Fallon, *Nourishing Traditions*, pp. xi–xii

Chapter Twelve

1. Michael Pollan, *In Defense of Food*, pg. 145 footnote
2. Ben Lerner, *Body by God*, pg. 53
3. Weston Price, *Nutrition and Physical Degeneration*, pg. 25
4. Jordan Rubin, *Patient, Heal Thyself*, pg. 45
5. James Trager, *The Food Chronology*, year 1944
6. William Dufty, *Sugar Blues*, pg. 61

Chapter Thirteen

1. William Wordsworth, English poet
2. William Wordsworth "rewritten for our time" by unknown author
3. Albert Wolters, *Creation Regained*, pg. 77
4. Joseph Mercola, *Dr. Mercola's Total Health Program*, pg. 255
5. Rex Russell, *What the Bible Says about Healthy Living*, pg. 234
6. William Dufty, *Sugar Blues*, pg. 213
7. Bruce Fife, *The Coconut Oil Miracle*, pg. 108

8. David Alan Black, "In Praise of Southern Agrarianism," http://www.freerepublic.com, February 2003

Chapter Fourteen

1. Jonathan Raban, author
2. Jordan Rubin, *The Maker's Diet*, pg. 290
3. Don Colbert, *What You Don't Know May Be Killing You*, pg. 58
4. Debra Lynn Dadd, *Home Safe Home*, pp. 15, 17–18
5. Don Colbert, *What You Don't Know May Be Killing You*, pp. 206–207
6. Ibid, pg. 59
7. Joseph Mercola, *Dr. Mercola's Total Health Program*, pg. 51
8. Don Colbert, *What You Don't Know May Be Killing You*, pg. 68
9. M.T. Whitney, "Mobile phones boost brain tumor risk by up to 270 percent on side of brain where phone is held," www.naturalnews.com, February 2007
10. Sue Kovach, "The Hidden Dangers of Cell Phone Radiation," www.lef.org/magazine/mag2007, August 2007
11. Christopher Babayode, "Wave your Health Good-Bye with Sky High WiFi," www.naturalnews.com, August 2009
12. Debra Lynn Dadd, *Home Safe Home*, pg. 19
13. Don Colbert, *What You Don't Know May Be Killing You*, pg. 224

Chapter Fifteen

1. Thomas Jefferson, U.S. President
2. G. Edward Griffin, *World Without Cancer*, pg. 53
3. Ibid. pg. xv
4. Sally Fallon, *Nourishing Traditions*, pg. 3
5. Ibid.
6. Dr. Ron Paul, "Protecting Health Freedom," www.lewrockwell.com, July 2007
7. Tracy Planinz, "Will Obama's new food czar end organic farming?" http://www.examiner.com, August 2009
8. Joel Salatin, *Holy Cows and Hog Heaven*, pg. 98
9. G. Edward Griffin, *World Without Cancer*, pg. 346
10. Benjamin Woolley, *Heal Thyself*, pgs. 125, 126
11. Ibid. pg. 141
12. Ibid. pg. 351
13. Ibid. pg. 352

14. Ibid. pg. 293
15. Ibid. pg. 351

Chapter Sixteen

1. Steve Meyerowitz, *The Organic Food Guide*, pg. 75
2. Joel Salatin, *Holy Cows and Hog Heaven*, pg. xv
3. Steve Meyerowitz, *The Organic Food Guide*, pg. 75
4. Michael Pollan, *In Defense of Food*, pg. 184
5. Steve Meyerowitz, *The Organic Food Guide*, pg. 9
6. Joel Salatin, *Holy Cows and Hog Heaven*, pp. 68–71
7. Michael Pollan, *In Defense of Food*, pg. 187
8. Karey Swan, *Hearth and Home*, pg. 12
9. Joel Salatin, *Holy Cows and Hog Heaven*, pg. 72
10. Azure Standard, an Oregon-based wholesale delivery company
11. Michael Pollan, *In Defense of Food*, pg. 158
12. Joel Salatin, *Holy Cows and Hog Heaven*, pg. 99
13. Ibid, pg. 6
14. Ibid. pg. 60
15. Ibid. pg. 64
16. Steve Meyerowitz, *The Organic Food Guide*, pg. 3
17. Ibid. pgs. 32,33
18. Ibid. pg. 57
19. Ibid. pg. 69
20. www.ediblecommunities.com

Chapter Seventeen

1. Shane Heaton, Australian nutritionist
2. Annie Eicher, "Organic Agriculture: A Glossary of Terms for Farmers and Gardeners" U.C. Davis, http://ucce.ucdavis.edu/files/filelibrary/1068/8268.pdf, February 2003.
3. Jordan Rubin, *Patient, Heal Thyself*, pp. 45
4. Joel Salatin, *Holy Cows and Hog Heaven*, pp. 54–55
5. Paul Fassa, "Why and how to avoid GMO foods," http://www.naturalnews.com, October 2009
6. Ibid.
7. Annie Eicher, "Organic Agriculture: A Glossary of Terms for Farmers and Gardeners" U.C. Davis, http://ucce.ucdavis.edu/files/filelibrary/1068/8268.pdf, February 2003

8. Steve Meyerowitz, *The Organic Food Guide*, pg. 37
9. Annie Eicher, "Organic Agriculture: A Glossary of Terms for Farmers and Gardeners" U.C. Davis, http://ucce.ucdavis.edu/files/filelibrary/1068/8268.pdf, February 2003
10. Ed Bauman, *Eating for Health*, pg. 32
11. Robert L. Wolke, "What's Natural?," Washington Post Online, May 2004
12. William Dufty, *Sugar Blues*, pg. 50
13. William Dufty, *Sugar Blues*, pg. 144
14. Don Colbert, *What You Don't Know May Be Killing You*, pg. 56
15. Steve Meyerowitz, *The Organic Food Guide*, pg. 36

Chapter Eighteen

1. Anonymous
2. Hippocrates, the father of medicine, quoted in *Nourishing Traditions*, pg. 479
3. Jordan Rubin, *Patient, Heal Thyself*, pg. 121
4. Sally Fallon, *Nourishing Traditions*, pgs. 26, 28, 31
5. Jordan Rubin, *The Maker's Diet*, pgs. 101, 103
6. Michel Montignac, *The French Diet*, pg. 94
7. Ibid. pp. 91
8. Ibid. pp. 8, 16
9. Ibid. pg. 30
10. Jordan Rubin, *Patient, Heal Thyself*, pg. 113
11. Jane Kinderlehrer, *Confessions of a Sneaky Organic Cook*, pg. 59

Chapter Nineteen

1. Renee DeGroot
2. Michel Montignac, *The French Diet*, pp. 32–35
3. Ibid. pg. 19
4. Jonny Bowden, *The 150 Healthiest Foods on Earth*, pg. 178
5. Michael Pollan, *In Defense of Food*, pg. 143
6. Bruce Fife, *The Coconut Oil Miracle*, pg. 27
7. Karey Swan, *Hearth and Home*, pg. 134
8. Jordan Rubin, *Patient, Heal Thyself*, pg. 142
9. Ray Strand and Bill Ewing, *Living By Design*, pg. 148
10. Michel Montignac, *The French Diet*, pg. 10
11. William Dufty, *Sugar Blues*, pg. 182
12. Headlines from www.naturalnews.com, September 2009 search

13. Joseph Mercola, *Dr. Mercola's Total Health Program*, pg. 51
14. Don Colbert, *What You Don't Know May Be Killing You*, pg. 26
15. Joseph Mercola, "Is Drinking Tea or Coffee the Smarter Choice?," www.articles. mercola.com, November 2009
16. Joseph Mercola, *Dr. Mercola's Total Health Program*, pg. 13
17. Rex Russell, *What the Bible Says About Healthy Living*, pp. 224–227

Chapter Twenty

1. Don Colbert, medical doctor
2. Don Colbert, *What You Don't Know May Be Killing You*, pg. 167
3. Bruce Fife, *The Coconut Oil Miracle*, pp. 25–26
4. Ibid. pg. 50
5. Ray Strand and Bill Ewing, *Living By Design*, pp. 126
6. Don Colbert, *What You Don't Know May Be Killing You*, pp. 106–107
7. Ibid.
8. Ben Lerner, *Body By God*, from pp. 51–53

Chapter Twenty-one

1. Annita Manning, medical reporter
2. Ed Bauman, *Eating for Health*, pg. 32
3. Joel Salatin, *Pastured Poultry Profits*, pg. 14
4. James Trager, *The Food Chronology*, years 1900–1995
5. Sally Fallon, *Nourishing Traditions*, pg. 25
6. Jane Kinderlehrer, *Confessions of a Sneaky Organic Cook*, pp. 55, 61
7. Jordan Rubin, *Patient, Heal Thyself*, pg. 135
8. Ibid.
9. Bruce Fife, *The Coconut Oil Miracle*, pg. 33
10. Jar label, Bragg Raw Unfiltered Organic Apple Cider Vinegar
11. James Trager, *The Food Chronology*, years 1967 and 1974
12. PPNF Health Journal quoted in *Nourishing Traditions*, pg. 551
13. James Trager, *The Food Chronology*, year 1952
14. William Dufty, *Sugar Blues*, pg. 60
15. James Trager, *The Food Chronology*, year 1952
16. William Dufty, *Sugar Blues*, pg. 149
17. Diane Campbell, *Step-by-Step to Natural Foods*, pg. 125

18. James Trager, *The Food Chronology*, year 1981
19. www.feingold.org/strawberry.html
20. Joel Salatin, *Holy Cows and Hog Heaven*, pg. 17
21. Sally Fallon, *Nourishing Traditions*, pg. 32
22. Sally Fallon, "Splendor from the Grass," Weston A. Price Foundation online
23. Ibid.
24. James Trager, *The Food Chronology*, years 1990–1995
25. Joel Salatin, *Holy Cows and Hog Heaven*, pg. 98
26. Ibid. pg 10
27. Ibid, pg. 30
28. Joel Salatin, *Salad Bar Beef*, pg. 242

Chapter Twenty-two

1. Ancient Chinese proverb
2. Luddene Perry, *A Field Guide to Buying Organic*, pg. 4

Chapter Twenty-three

1. Thomas Edison, inventor
2. Terry A. Rondberg, *Chiropractic First*, pg. 24
3. Jordan Rubin, *The Maker's Diet*, pg. 259
4. Sally Fallon, *Nourishing Traditions*, pg. 620
5. Ray Strand and Bill Ewing, *Living By Design*, pg. 145
6. Barbara Minton, "Sleep May be the Critical Factor for Weight Loss and Health," www.naturalnews.com, January 2009
7. Jordan Rubin, *The Maker's Diet*, pp. 83,159
8. Ibid. pg. 55

Chapter Twenty-four

1. Michael Pollan, *In Defense of Food*, pg. 200
2. Psalm 107:31–39; Proverbs 31:14–16; Isaiah 1:19–20; 18:4–6; 58:11; 61:11; Jeremiah 29:5
3. Jonny Bowden, *The 150 Healthiest Foods on Earth*, pp. 14–15

Chapter Twenty-five

1. John Locke, philosopher
2. Joel Salatin, *Holy Cows and Hog Heaven*, pg. 124

Chapter Twenty-six

1. Old Hundredth Psalm, William Kethe

While all of the included quotations and citations are believed to be *fair use* based on accepted literary standards, permission was requested from and granted by the following authors or their agents.

Quotations from Don Colbert, Debra Lynn Dadd, Sally Fallon, Bruce Fife, Joseph Mercola, Michel Montignac, Steve Meyerowitz, Michael Pollan, Joel Salatin, Ray Strand, Jordan Rubin, and Benjamin Woolley are used with express permission.

PW

Breinigsville, PA USA
22 October 2010
247901BV00003B/25/P